NATURAL BABYCARE

PURE AND SOOTHING RECIPES AND TECHNIQUES FOR MOTHERS AND BABIES

COLLEEN K. DODT

STOREY
BOOKS
Schoolhouse Road
Pownal, Vermont 05261

The mission of Storey Communications is to serve our customers by publishing practical information that encourages personal independence in harmony with the environment.

Edited by Deborah L. Balmuth
Cover design by Carol J. Jessop, Black Trout Design and Meredith Maker
Cover illustration and spot art © John Nelson/Represented by Irmeli Holmberg
Text design by Carol J. Jessop, Black Trout Design
Text production by Susan Bernier
Line drawings by Laura Tedeschi except for pages 28, 29, and 74 by
    Brigita Fuhrmann
Indexed by Word•a•bil•ity

Printed in the United States by R. R. Donnelley
10 9 8 7 6 5 4 3 2

Library of Congress Cataloging-in-Publication Data

Dodt, Colleen K., 1955–
        Natural babycare : pure and soothing recipes and techniques for mothers and
    babies / Colleen K. Dodt
                p.   cm.
        Includes bibliographical references.
        ISBN 0-88266-953-2 (pbk. : alk. paper)
        1. Infants—Care.   2. Prenatal care.   3. Naturopathy.   4. Holistic medicine.
        I. Title
    RJ61.D625   1997
    649'.122—dc20   96-46122
                                                                                CIP

TABLE OF CONTENTS

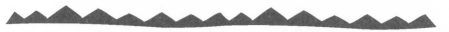

INSPIRATION

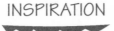

To Christina and David Dodt, the wonderful children I have been honored to directly share my life with, and all of the other children God has entrusted to my care and attention whether through my love, a book, a garden, a hug, a look, a scent, a flower, an herb, or a mother's inspiration to care for them in the most natural fashion possible through the mother earth and all of her abundance.

Thank you Gary, my herbal treasure.

Sue, I wish a mother's peace.

A flowerbed for Sandy so she can rest.

For George, an herbal bouquet and a splash of rosewater.

To the unseen hands that guide, my deepest respect and gratitude.

Special thanks to the companies that shared information on their products or concepts and toil to make the world a little better for the children we love.

Let us teach each and every child that rain does indeed often yield to rainbows.

Let us inspire them to live life to its fullest and always to believe in themselves by believing in our own selves and our ability to gently guide these precious children entrusted into our care. Remember the child alive in your heart.

Had the eyes no tears, the soul would have no rainbows.

I share with you a page from Christina's book, a book I have been writing since before her conception.

June 4, 1986

My Sweet Child,

You sleep in a peaceful rest. I just got up to put on paper how much I adore you, Christina. After you fell asleep to a lovely tape of harp music, I kissed you, hugged you, wished you peace and cried for Love of you. I want you to know you are a precious child and mean life to me.

My thanks, sweet being.

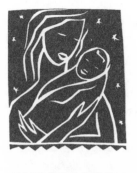

INTRODUCTION

The moment that I learned I was expecting a child was one of the happiest of my life. I had always wondered if I would have kids and, if I did, what they would look and be like. The realization that I was responsible for another human being hit me with a desire to give this child and myself the very best nature has to offer. Coincidentally, that same day I received in the mail a catalog from an herb company. I had always had an interest in natural ways; this new stage of my life was the motivation I needed to delve into an apprenticeship to mother earth with zeal.

I read everything I could find on holistic ways and experimented eagerly, often with amazing results. It was as though I already knew the herbs, essential oils, and homeopathic remedies I encountered. I had a natural ability to learn and teach the ways of these precious products. I believe many of you do, too. A number of these ways are ancient, perhaps part of our ancestral memory. Many have been in practice throughout centuries of healing, and were recorded and passed on in day books from mother to daughter.

LEARNING FROM THE WISDOM OF TIMES PAST

One interesting account of the evolution of herbal healing and medicines is presented in *Green Pharmacy: A History of Herbal Medicine* by Barbara Griggs. She relates how herbs have been an intimate part of human households throughout history. Some of the things used to heal were frightening (by today's standards), some sublime. Concoctions prepared by elaborate apothecaries were often expensive and contained some very disagreeable ingredients. The seemingly more useful medicines, according to Griggs, were those developed by learned housewives from materials gathered from nearby hedgerows or countryside fields.

In a chapter entitled "The Seventeenth-Century Super-woman," Griggs describes the tasks a woman of that period performed and the knowledge she was required to have just to maintain a household. She was often brewer, baker, doctor, and farmer rolled into one. Neighbors and the community also depended on her expertise. Children were often lost as a result of unskilled hands. Learning the ways of healing with herbs was not a choice but a direct necessity of survival. This knowl-edge was passed down by word-of-mouth or by carefully main-tained receipt books. A degree of healing knowledge is still important to acquire today. You and your family can benefit from the herbal healing wisdom of times past.

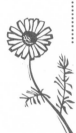

Another book from Barbara Griggs, *The Green Witch Herbal: Restoring Nature's Magic in Home, Health, and Beauty*, includes a wealth of information and suggestions for how to incorporate healing herbs into your life. She has a good chapter on "Herbal Remedies For Children" that covers colic, colds, fever, and a useful first aid section. Cooking with herbs, bathing, skin care, and how to prepare herbal remedies are also covered.

ALTERNATIVE OPTIONS

People of the seventeenth century faced with life-and-death decisions had to rely only on their ability to recognize and know the uses of medicinal plants and remedies. Today, we are fortunate to have a variety of healthcare options open to us, from high-tech hospitals to alternative-medicine techniques. We have the freedom to select and use alternative techniques in ways we feel comfortable with to complement our overall healthcare plan.

Some of the alternative remedies are complicated to under-stand, but most of them are easy. Nature's gentle healers have come to my rescue numerous times. I have subjected these techniques to extensive examination and questioning, and am pleased to be able to share the results of my inquiries. You, too, can acquire a simple working knowledge of several herbs, oils, and homeopathic remedies. This basic "alternative" education will save you sleepless nights and extra medical bills, and enable you to teach your family the gentle art of taking care of each other.

Natural home remedies are not a replacement for traditional medical care, but they can be a complement to preventative healthcare and to follow-up home care to help a family member heal.

Being involved in your children's care, no matter what their ages, is a powerful way to enhance their wellness. To stand passively by while others administer care to our kids can be a very difficult thing to do. We are intimately connected to our children, to all children. We are the ones they trust and the ones under whose care they will usually best flourish. Proper and competent medical care is always a must and I wouldn't suggest treating a child solely with home remedies. However, some simple little things we can do for them can greatly enhance and support any other care they must receive, and often prevent further problems.

We influence children's health from before conception and throughout their lives. The habits we keep ourselves will be visited back upon us as we watch our children become parents. We set the stage for how our children view life, and the associations we instill in them will be carried throughout life. I have told my own lovely daughter Christina, who is exactly 25 years younger than I, that even if she were 75 and I were 100, she would still be my baby!

We want the best of everything for these little folks that we have been entrusted with, and through natural baby and child-care practices we can show them how much they mean to us, and enhance everything from their diets to their immune systems. Note I said "practices." We are all practicing. No one will ever be perfect at caring for a child, yet with nature's bounty of herbs, pure essential oils, and homeopathic remedies we can help launch them into a healthy future.

MY BACKGROUND AND APPROACH

When I first began experimenting with pure essential oils back in 1980, I didn't realize that I was headed on an aromatic journey that would last a lifetime. Like many other folks my age, my main experience with pure essential oils was patchouli oil in the '60s. Sandalwood and a bit of lavender were all I knew of aromatherapy, and it would take a few years of acquaintance with herbs before I became intrigued with what makes them smell as they do.

Pure essential oils got my attention every time I gently squeezed an herbal sachet. Peeling an orange for a snack or crushing lavender flowers for a bath released these precious substances for me to savor. As I would pass by the clary sage and hyssop plants flowering in the gardens, my skirt would gather the pure essential oils and release them to me later as I sat in the sun. I wondered what it was that made me feel so invigorated when I rinsed my hair with fresh sprigs of rosemary and basil made into an infusion. Or what was so soothing about my rose, lavender, and chamomile herbal bath. While sipping a warm cup of spearmint or peppermint tea, my nose would tingle in delight.

Every time I took a child through my scratch-and-sniff gardens I was beckoned to acquire more knowledge about the marvelous essences that make the scented leaves of lemon balm and rose geranium so fragrant.

Why did crushed eucalyptus leaves, when combined with thyme and peppermint, bring relief when I was feeling congested? Why did the exotic scents of my tuberose seem so intoxicating as it bloomed near my door? And what about that tart oil that was squeezed into my hand when I crushed a lemon wedge into a glass of spring water? Why did the redolent smoke from my brass burner filled with frankincense and myrrh make my prayers seem more sacred and my breathing deeper and stronger?

Discovering Aromatherapy

In 1985, I found a book entitled *The Art of Aromatherapy* by Robert Tisserand, and this gave me the first really concrete knowledge on the precious substances I would come to know as pure essential oils. The term "Aromatherapy" explained what I had been doing with my herbs for many years and helped me gain insight into how to use just the pure essential oils of herbs, flowers, barks, and resins. I was in aromatic heaven. After contacting Tisserand, I visited him in England to ask more about this wonderful new art. I came home with a passion for the aromatic spirits of plants, a collection of pure essential oils, and a mission — to do my part to aromatize America.

I had the honour of being the first American woman to be featured in *The International Journal of Aromatherapy,* edited by Robert Tisserand out of England, and my company, Herbal Endeavours Ltd., was the first company in America to bring him here to teach. I was inspired to share the knowledge with as many people as possible. I began to search out like-minded people. I have experienced many reactions to herbalism and aromatherapy, as you could imagine, in the last 10 years. Some think it's the most wonderful thing they have ever discovered; others call me a witch or an old hippie who can't get a real job.

Aromatherapy, American-Style

I have seen aromatherapy associations come and go. I have tried to reach some for information on membership only to have my phone call go unanswered. Other groups left it unclear what I would receive for my membership fee. We as aromatherapy consultants are where the massage therapists were a decade ago: unorganized, yet working very hard at getting there. We will all experience growing pains. I don't know where aromatherapy stands legally in any of the states, but I am aware of no set standards; much still depends upon personal ethics. So rather than get involved with the politics of business, I set out to teach one soul at a time how to safely incorporate pure essential oils into her life. I teach in small community education classes, senior citizen centers, at craft shows, in my garden, and anywhere that I am asked about that wonderful scent that travels as a part of me. I often smile when a bank teller says, "Your deposits smell so good." "I don't scent them," I reply, "they just live with me in my aromatic household."

AROMATHERAPIST?

I have struggled with what to call myself and my aromatic endeavors. I don't feel I am an aromatherapist in the way the British use the term. I blend oils and consult, but do not touch my clients through massage. (I send them to a massage therapist.) I don't care for the term "aromatic consultant" because that just sounds like I am a consultant who smells aromatic. I do use "aroma consultant" and "creator of pure high-quality herbal and aromatherapy products."

Mine is a small cottage business, yet I have reached far and wide with my sweetly scented message. Letters come from South Africa, Colombia, Singapore, Peru, Finland, England, China, Japan, Germany, and Jamaica, to name just some. I have seen students leave a class on personal perfume blending clutching a small amber bottle as if it were gold.

HOW A TEACHER IS TAUGHT

In my career I have been taught more than I could ever teach. Each student, client, and customer brings her own personal view of aromatherapy and how it works for her.

I had the honor of being one of the first aromatherapy teachers to address an international conference, in Louisville, Kentucky, in 1988 and in San Jose, California, in 1989. The response was amazing. People who previously had dismissed aromatherapy sat up and listened, and now love the oils as I do.

Herbs, pure essential oils, homeopathic remedies, massage, organic foods, music, and Bach flower remedies, used properly and with caution, can make a difference for you, your kids, and the whole world. I invite you to read this book with an open mind, a willingness to explore, and a determination to provide the best for your child and yourself. The farther you look back, the farther ahead you can see. Let us review some age-old practices of child-rearing and care. Use what works for you. This information is not to instill guilt in the way you currently approach child rearing; I wish only to offer you the best natural alternatives. Use the resource list; call or write to them today. Make this the day you opened your eyes and took time to stop and smell the flowers, perhaps with a very small hand in yours. As I write I hear neighbor children leaving lilacs at my back door. I have earned their respect and confidence from my genuine concern for their lives and well-being. Somehow, I just know . . . they know.

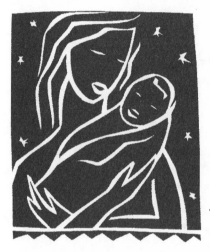

A Primer of
Natural-Care
Products and
Techniques

CHAPTER

By simply picking up this book you have made a choice to investigate the possibilities of using natural baby-care products and techniques. When anticipating the arrival of a baby or small child into your life, your thoughts will quite easily turn to questions such as:

◆ How will I know what is best for my child?
◆ What methods and products will I use to care for my child?
◆ Do so-called natural products work, are they safe to use, and are they economically feasible to use on a limited budget?
◆ Where can I find ready-to-use natural products that I can be assured of high quality?

This chapter will begin to provide answers to these questions by introducing you to some tried-and-true practices that can ease the responsibility of parenting and caring for the young. Let mother nature reveal her own personal recipes and resources to you. Partake in her natural abundance and know you are providing exceptional natural alternatives to your family and self.

HERBS

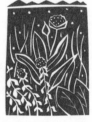 There is a renewed interest today in using herbs and herbal remedies for improving and maintaining children's health as well as adults'. Some companies are now offering ready-made herbal products for families who want to take advantage of them in their homes, yet lack the time to grow, study, or prepare them. Teas, tinctures, capsules, and salves can be valuable assets in any medicine chest (see page 96). Always consult a knowledgeable doctor or herbalist before administering any herbal remedy to a child.

Herbal therapy need not be shrouded in myth and mystery, nor perceived as weird or fanatical medicine. Simple herbal cures have been used and proven effective for centuries. Dill water was commonly administered in centuries past for colic, and mints have been used by many generations to ease indigestion, hydrate, and cool the body. With today's modern methods of scientific analysis, we know even more about these wondrous substances called herbs and how they interact with our bodies, minds, and spirits.

I recall providing Christina and her playmates with cool, refreshing lemonade in the heat of summer. Instead of tart lemons (that often require a lot of sugar to make them palatable), I used lemon balm and lemon verbena. Herbal teas are a great way to introduce your children to herbs. Offer them in place of soft drinks or the awful colored water so many children are accustomed to receiving. If they are given herbal teas on a consistent basis, children will not always associate herbs with ill health. Some healing herbs can taste nasty, though, so balancing them with tastier ones will better enable you to coax a small one to try them.

The essential oil content of the fresh and dried herbs is much less than the pure essential oils themselves, which are at 100 percent strength. Experiment with fresh and dried herbs to familiarize yourself with their scents, properties, and uses in a milder way. Oranges, lemons, and grapefruits contain essential oil in their peels, but they also may contain pesticides, so try to procure organic fruits whenever possible, especially when you're planning to use them in a tea.

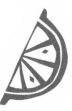

Herbal Tea

A simple rule of thumb for making an infusion (tea) is to steep 1 teaspoon of dried herbs in 1 cup of water for 5 to 10 minutes.

An infusion of peppermint or catnip sweetened with a little honey can work wonders to help quiet jangled nerves — Mom's or child's. Get in the habit of keeping some iced peppermint or lemon balm tea in the fridge and don't be surprised to see the kids reaching for that instead of a soda!

You can make a delicious tea with ginger. And if you add a little honey, you've got a wonderful soother for an upset stomach or a stuffy nose.

THE BENEFITS OF HERBAL TEAS

Getting yourself and family members to each drink eight glasses of water a day can be difficult. Herbs are just the thing to add life to water. They give it a wonderful refreshing taste and aroma. Even the herbs that aren't so tasty are, to say the least, interesting!

In the summer, I like to keep a pitcher of spearmint, lemon balm, and garden sage tea in the refrigerator. Its gentle green hue is much easier to drink than those dark, fuzzy, sickly sweet concoctions that are mass-marketed.

When you're brewing herb tea, make it a practice to prepare a pot rather than just one cup. This way you're likely to drink more and, if you have any left over, you can always feed it to your plants or use it as a hair rinse. You sure don't want to try *that* with one of the popular sugared beverages! Moreover, I put the spent herbs on my houseplants and garden to act as a mulch. Herb teas revive us deeply, and can be made a part of every household. Use what you grow; grow what you use.

Herbal Baths

An herbal or aromatherapy bath are two of life's finest pleasures. Many a crazy day was brought back to sanity with the simple addition of an aromatic bath. The relaxing warmth fills you as you lower your body into the scented vapors.

For a new parent, an herbal bath can provide much needed balance and relaxation. It is your time to be you. Take a few moments to allow the stress to release from your muscles and the mind to let go in the redolent warmth of the fragrant waters. I often took an herb bath when Christina was asleep or in an infant carrier seat. I would sit her on the floor of the bathroom and enjoy my own deeply relaxing, nurturing time. While she snoozed, I soothed. Some days I would bath her and put her down for a nap, and then go in to unwind in my own aromatherapy spa — my tub.

Foot Baths

When you don't have time or the inclination for a whole tub bath, a foot bath is a nice alternative. Simply add a few drops of pure essential oil or crushed dry or fresh herbs to a small tub of warm water. Follow up by applying an aromatic cream, lotion, or oil to your feet and putting on clean, warm, cotton socks. Foot baths are nice for the whole family . . . dad too!

One night, my 15-year-old nephew George and a young friend, Corey, whom I help care for, were doing their homework at my house. I suggested a foot bath would refresh them and help them to remember their lessons. My willing clients shed their shoes and thoroughly enjoyed the lemon, juniper, and rosemary foot bath.

COMMON HERBS TO HAVE ON HAND

Following are just a few of the common herbs that can enhance the well being of a household. Most can be grown in a home garden or easily obtained through the mail-order suppliers of herbs (see "Herbal Products" on page 146). There are many more medicinal herbs, Chinese herbs, rainforest herbs, and a multitude of others that await the willing explorer in this realm. There are many ways to find out more. Classes and publications on the topic of herbs and alternative healthcare are emerging in communities everywhere. Many nurses, doctors, and midwives are getting additional training in herbal and aromatic healing. Visit the holistic health or alternative medicine section of your favorite bookstore or library to discover some of the marvelous herbals available today.

MAKING AN HERBAL BATH

To create an herbal bath, first make a tea from fresh or dried herbs (as described on page 68) and then pour the tea through a strainer into a tubful of warm water.

It's also easy to make herbal bath salts by blending 1 tablespoon of chopped dried herbs with 1 pint of sea salt. Dried peppermint, rosemary, spearmint, lavender, roses, lemon balm, or lemon verbena all make great combinations. To use, add 2 tablespoons of salts to a tubful of warm water and enjoy.

Herbs should be stored in well-sealed dark glass bottles, preferably in a dark cupboard. Many herbs (especially those used for cooking) are kept above the stove where they are exposed to too much heat, light, and moisture which dissipate their essences. Store your herbs well and the reward will be freshly dried herbs in the middle of winter, just the thing for a winter bath or cup of tea.

CATNIP
Nature: This plant grows beautifully in the garden and re-seeds easily. The tea has been used for jangled nerves. I usually mix catnip with an equal amount of mint to dilute the strong taste.
Benefits: Soothes mild fevers and colic.

CHAMOMILE
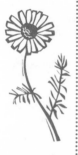
Nature: This small daisylike flower is ready to pick when the white petals fall back to resemble a great Indian chief's head-dress. Its calming influence has been noted by many. Chamomile has been favored for centuries as a hair rinse for light-colored hair. *Note:* Some people with allergies to ragweed and other plants may react to chamomile.
Benefits: Soothes mild fevers, colic, upset stomachs, headaches. Remember that Peter Rabbit's mother gave him chamomile tea.

CAUTION

Before using any medicinal herbs be sure to thoroughly research their potential effects, especially if you are pregnant. Some of the herbs contraindicated (advised against use) during pregnancy or breastfeeding include: bloodroot, blue cohosh (however, can be used at birth), ephedra, licorice, mandrake, mistletoe, pennyroyal, poke root, rue, sage, shepherd's purse(can be used at birth), tansy, thuja, and wormwood.

Herbs that have been found by some to be useful during pregnancy or breastfeeding include: fennel, ginger, and peppermint teas to ease morning sickness; dandelion root and yellow dock for building blood in iron-poor mothers. Obtain a reputable book on herbs for the childbearing years before taking anything (see reading list).

ECHINACEA

Nature: This herb comes in many varieties and merits further investigation for any home medicine chest. I have turned to echinacea at times when we were pretty sick with sore throat, flu, colds, and general immune weaknesses. Use caution with dosages for babies and/or children. I generally use it in a tincture form, although the alcohol is not appropriate for infants. Be sure to select a tincture made with organically grown herbs as the pesticides can be concentrated in a tincture.

Benefits: Echinacea is a general infection fighter, antiseptic, and immune stimulator.

FENNEL

Nature: Fennel is beautiful to grow. Its tall, feathery presence holds a prominent position over other herbs in the garden. The leaf, seed, and bulb are each used in a variety of ways, from chopped into a soup (the leaf) to chewed as an after-dinner treat (the seed). I love to pass by a tall fennel plant and bite off a few pungent seeds to soothe my stomach or freshen my breath. I often carry a few flower heads of seeds in my pocket.

Benefits: Soothes upset stomach and intestinal gas. Fennel tea is soothing after eating. Increases milk flow in nursing mothers.

GINGER

Nature: Available in most grocery stores and all specialty stores, ginger comes in several forms. The fresh root is best kept in the refrigerator. I also keep the powdered and fresh dried root forms.

Benefits: Soothes upset stomach, mild fevers, hives, intestinal gas, motion and morning sickness. Ginger has a warming effect.

A small dab (½ teaspoon) of powdered ginger added to a warm bathtub can be quite comforting to a child suffering from itchy chicken pox.

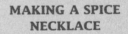

MAKING A SPICE NECKLACE

One way I enjoy keeping the scent of rich, fragrant spices like ginger close at hand is to make a spice necklace. I string the dried ginger root, along with whole cloves, cinnamon sticks, star anise, and allspice berries on a strong piece of waxed cotton or twine using a large-holed needle. The interesting shapes of dried ginger root make it very useful as a central piece in the necklace.

LEMON BALM

Nature: This is the first herb I remember learning to identify, aside from the fresh dandelion greens my neighbor old Mary picked in her front yard when I was a young girl. I found lemon balm growing along the walls of my neighbor Sue's house and wondered what it was. Its scent and flavor is lovely and lemony. Melissa is its other name; the essential oil is costly and rare although the herb is prolific in most gardens. A tea of this herb is unbeatable to refresh and soothe. Dry some in small bunches for winter use.

Benefits: Soothes mild fevers, fights infection, relaxes.

LEMONGRASS

Nature: I am happy when I can obtain a plant of this grass, which is great in soups, teas, or as a refreshing bath. The pure essential oil has an intense pungency; I prefer the fresh or dried plant. The plant can be grown in a pot, but needs to be brought inside for the winter.

Benefits: Soothes mild fevers, fights infection, anti-viral, refreshing.

PEPPERMINT

Nature: Freshly harvested peppermint is a pungent delight. Whether being used in a refreshing tea or a cooling herb bath, peppermint cannot be beat to refresh and cool. I dry this herb for winter use in tea for an upset stomach or just to dispel winter's chill. The warm scent is opening, clear, and uplifting. For a lightly cooling bath salt, try blending 1 tablespoon chopped dried peppermint with 1 pint sea salt. The minute amount of pure essential oils present in the freshly crushed leaves of the freshly dried herb peppermint when added to the sea salt is just enough.

Benefits: Soothes stomach, relieves intestinal gas, mild fevers, headaches, fights infection. Refreshing, uplifting, and opening.

CAUTION

Peppermint essential oil must be used with extreme caution! I seldom employ this essential oil. It is very potent and much too intense for babies or young children.

SPEARMINT

Nature: This herb is quite different from peppermint and equally as refreshing. I think of spearmint as a bit more refined. A tea or herb bath with spearmint is refreshing and uplifting. It combines well with lavender, and roses for a bath. Spearmint should definitely be used often fresh in the summer, and dried for winter use. When you're growing either peppermint or spearmint, be sure to obtain high-quality cuttings. Rather than accept the strange varieties they offer in many nurseries, ask a gardener for a cutting of authentic peppermint or spearmint.

Benefits: Soothes stomach upset, relieves gas and morning sickness, makes a refreshing herbal water or herb bath.

WRITE IT ALL DOWN

This poem was presented to me by a dear friend, Mr. G. I give it to you to remind you to record your own personal aromatic experiences. When you develop an herb blend you particularly like, write it down. I have lost blends that I just was so sure I knew by heart. Record, experiment, and take time to stop and smell the roses, lavender, rosemary, bergamot . . .

The pleasure a writer knows
is the pleasure of sages
Out of non-being, being is born;
out of silence, a writer produces a song.
In the yard of silk, there is infinite space;
language is a deluge from one small corner of the heart.
The net of images is cast wider and wider;
thought searches more and more deeply.
The writer offers a fragrance of fresh flowers
an abundance of sprouting buds.
Bright winds lift each metaphor,
clouds lift from a forest of writing brushes.

— Lu Chi

Resources for Learning More

Healing Children Naturally by Michael A. Weiner, Ph.D., is a "must-have" title for any parent's library (see reading list on page 151). It is an A to Z of natural approaches for a variety of complaints, a comprehensive guide to sensible treatments for many childhood ailments.

Nutrition during pre-conception, pregnancy, lactation, and the first years of a child's life are crucially important to a lifetime of good health. Foods can be one of our greatest healing allies. When proper nutrition is observed, many ailments are of short duration or even short circuited. In today's prepackaged world, nutrition is often taken for granted. I see some food products in the store and wonder how companies can be allowed to sell them to the public. Many are laden with additives and ingredients that have little or no nutritional value to our lives.

In his book, Dr. Weiner addresses nutritional issues as well as simple herbal remedies for many of the everyday situations we are faced with during child rearing. In a clear, straightforward manner, Dr. Weiner explains how diet can help address the health needs of children who are prone to allergies, asthma, bed-wetting, colds, flu, earache, Sudden Infant Death Syndrome (SIDS), insomnia, and milk intolerance. He includes recipes for meals addressing your child's particular healthcare needs. Weiner also provides a nice overview of ethnic and cultural dietary differences.

Herbal preparations can be a valuable supplement to your child's diet. Dr. Weiner offers some simple guidelines for incorporating Mother Nature's lovely herbs in your child's meals. Two of the easiest ways to use fresh and dried herbs are in a tea (an infusion) or an herbal bath. Both have many healing properties.

ESSENTIAL OILS

 Everyday, my mailbox is full with requests for more information on life's essentials, pure essential oils. They have aided me in the birth and the death of loved ones. They have held my heart in gentle rose-scented hands when times were rough.

ESSENTIAL OILS IN THE BATH

For a foot bath made with essential oils, add 1 drop each of three selected oils (or 6 drops of one oil) to 2 gallons warm water and mix well. The essential oils may also be diluted in base oil, milk or cream, or sea salt before being added to the water, if desired.

You can also make up a jar of foot bath salts in advance, label it well, and keep it on hand for those days when just getting a basin of hot water poured is a challenge! Sea salt is a great base for bath salts and helps make your precious, costly oils go further. You only need 1 or 2 drops to 2 cups of sea salt. I like to combine coarse and fine grinds. Sea salt is soothing to soak in and looks lovely when some small amounts of herbs or flowers are added to it, along with the pure essential oils and absolutes. Keep these precious crystals well stoppered! When you're ready to use them, add 2 tablespoons of the salts (or dried herbs) to the tub of water for quick relief. (*Note:* Pregnant women should always exercise caution in using essential oils.)

They have let me rest upon lavender-scented pillows, and provided a soothing aromatherapy massage for aching muscles after a long day of gardening. Pure essential oils have kept my body, mind, and spirit in balance. They offer these benefits to all humankind; if you only let them.

Pure essential oils and absolutes are very concentrated. Therefore, only small amounts need be used or applied to gain results. Many pounds of herbs, flowers, or resins and fruits are used in the production of only small amounts of oils. *Less is best* is what I tell my work-study students and clients. Many people think that if two drops of an oil will help them feel better, more oil will lead to greater relaxation, or stimulation — not so! Sometimes using too much essential oils can actually have a boomerang effect and aggravate symptoms.

Essential oils can be expensive, and using less is smart economically, as well.

Use in Dilution

Pure essential oils are almost always used in dilution, very seldom are they used "neat." (Neat doesn't mean they are "cool";

it's a term used to mean "undiluted or straight.") Tea tree, sandalwood, patchouli, and jasmine and rose absolute have never given me a problem being used neat. Lavender is one oil I feel confident in using neat. I dab it on small cuts, scrapes, burns, bumps, and insect bites.

Most other essential oils I use in a dilution of sweet almond oil (see "Dilutions and Solutions" on page 30) or some other base or carrier oil like grapeseed, apricot kernel, or jojoba *(ha-ho-ba)*, which is actually a liquid wax. I also add the oils to a high-quality, unscented cream or lotion base for use on my skin when I don't want to be too oily.

Purchasing Essential Oils

Buyer beware! Many companies make a lot of money from the sale of pure essential oils, and just as many make money from the sale of inferior products they *call* pure essential oils. I fear this will get worse before it gets better. There are no established guidelines for products as of this writing.

My advice to potential essential oil purchasers is "Buyer beware"; better yet, "Let the buyer be educated." Synthetic aromatic chemicals fill our very existence. Many so-called essential oils have been reconstituted or diluted. The temptation is just too much for some businesses to resist.

High-quality essential oils can be quite costly. Purchase them as you use them, and if there is an oil that is out of your financial range, ask some friends if they would like to share an order. Remember, most oils are diluted in a carrier oil, and a few small drops will go a very long way.

Pure essential oils must be respected, researched, and worked with to truly understand them. Start with one or two oils and get to know them intimately. Be specific about your needs, and research the oils that can be of greatest assistance to achieve your desired outcomes. Obtain reliable books, subscribe to a journal or magazine, research and join an organization, experiment with someone who has some experience and time to play. Whenever possible, consult a qualified aromatherapist, consultant, naturopathic doctor, or an M.D. with an interest in aromatherapy.

Midwives are becoming much more knowledgeable in the art of aromatherapy, and may be able to suggest pure essential oils that have aided their clients or themselves. Pure essential oils are worth the time and expense necessary to get to know them.

Interest now is toward more organically grown and wild-crafted (harvested in the wild) oils and those from small independent distillers. I support this wholeheartedly and hope it continues. However, I object to essential oil companies that get caught up in being the best, the richest, or the most difficult to understand by constantly introducing rare and exotic oils.

ESSENTIAL OILS SAFETY TIPS

◆ Buy the highest-quality essential oils available to you (I use lesser-quality oils to wash my floors, but never my body).

◆ Dispense by the drop, carefully, and count. Record your recipes accurately.

◆ Less is best. Dilute, dilute, dilute. Resist the urge to use more. Pure essential oils are very seldom used "neat," or undiluted, on the skin, with the exception of tea tree and lavender. I have used other oils neat but this is subject to individual skin sensitivity. Do a patch test on the inside of the arm to determine how you will react. Pure essential oils like cinnamon, clove, juniper, and some citrus can be very irritating. Exercise caution if you will be exposed to the sun when using bergamot and other citrus oils.

◆ Use cotton swabs or cotton buds to apply pure essential oils; hands and fingers may eventually contaminate the bottle. Dropper-top bottles easily dispense a drop at a time, making it less likely that you will use too much essential oil or accidentally have a spill.

◆ Wipe your essential oil bottles clean. Be careful where you set them; essential oils can mar surfaces, especially plastic ones. Always make sure bottle caps are twisted on securely.

◆ Practice aromatic etiquette. Many scents may be perceived as offensive to others. Use essential oils and perfumes in moderation in public, and check with family members to make sure your precious vapors aren't causing anyone else distress because of allergies, asthma, or just personal preference.

◆ Label everything — for your own convenience and others' safety. Clearly label and put away from children any potentially harmful substances. (Labeling is a great chance to be creative, too.)

My goal is to enlighten the average person on the everyday use of pure essential oils, to help you replace the aromatic impostors with pure essential oils. This is what I term "home aroma." The use of essential oils does not require special training or special occasions. If you are interested in learning about the hundreds of ways you can introduce essential oils into your everyday home environment, you may enjoy *The Essential Oils Book* (see reading list).

PRECAUTIONS AND CAUTIONS

Working with pure essential oils can be rewarding in a number of ways. It can also be dangerous when precautions and cautions aren't properly observed. Everyone is different and will react to individual essential oils in various manners. Some simple precautions will make your experiences much more pleasant.

Keep Out of the Reach of Children

Pure essential oils can be toxic if ingested in large amounts and harmful to the skin and eyes if spilled or improperly undiluted. Children never should play with oils. I have had phone calls from kids who were using oils when their parents were away from home. I was happy they sought help, but distressed that they were left to experiment on their own!

Whether to use oils on babies is debatable. Some sources say yes; some no. I would not use them on an infant without proper supervision and direction. I have seen beneficial results with using oils in children as young as two and successfully employed them with my own daughter over the years. She is now 16 and still uses them when needed.

Use Caution During Pregnancy

While some people advise against using any essential oils during pregnancy, other books offer detailed advise on how to use the oils in a limited way during this time. I advise extreme caution, particularly during the first trimester since some findings indicate a potential danger of developmental defects and increased risk of miscarriage. Many oils can stimulate the uterus. This may be a great effect to encourage as birth approaches, but, obviously, it is not desirable at two months into the pregnancy. I have attended births where pure essentials were used along with jasmine absolute to assist in the birthing process with marvelous results. If you are interested in this possibility, I advise working with a doctor, midwife, or aromatherapist who specializes in this area. Some essential oil specialists have also reported success in using a combination of pure essential oils and very high-quality carrier oils, applied faithfully after the third month of pregnancy, to reduce stretch marks.

Essential oils that I advise avoiding during pregnancy include: basil, cedarwood, cinnamon, clary sage, clove, cypress, fennel, hyssop, jasmine, juniper, lemongrass, myrrh, parsley, pennyroyal, peppermint, rose, rosemary, sweet marjoram, thyme. Avoid chamomile, geranium, lavender, melissa, and sage during the first three months; use after that time with caution.

Never Use These Oils

Toxicity can occur with regular use of bitter almond, calamus, cassia (cinnamon leaf), cinnamon, clove, mugwort, pennyroyal, sassafras, tansy, thuja, thyme, wintergreen, wormwood.

Thoroughly research any and all essential oil before use!

COMMON ESSENTIAL OILS

ROMAN CHAMOMILE (*Chamaemelum nobile*)
GERMAN CHAMOMILE (*Matricaria recutita*)
Nature: Roman chamomile and German chamomile are distilled from certain types of chamomile flower. Roman is clear and sweet; German is usually a deep blue-green and has a much more bitter scent.
Benefits: Believed to be analgesic, anti-inflammatory, antispasmodic, and a nerve sedative.
Suggestions for use: This oil is a must for headache sufferers. It has helped me through some rough ones when all other oils have failed. I apply 2 drops in a bowl of warm water, press an absorbent cloth (cloth diaper would work fine) to the top of the water, fold it, and apply it to my forehead (exercise caution near eyes with all essential oils). Two drops of lavender is a nice

addition to a compress. I also have added this oil to a water spray with lavender for sunburn. Use 2 drops Roman chamomile, German chamomile, or yarrow and 5 drops of lavender. Apply liberally.

As a before-bed bath, it is unsurpassed to help a person unwind, much as the herbal tea of German chamomile has been used for centuries. There are a few types of chamomile. Get to know each one individually and thoroughly.

This is a potent yet mild pure essential oil. It can be expensive; fortunately, very little is needed. It smells fresh and clean.

CLARY SAGE (Salvia sclarea)
Benefits: Clary sage has been found to be anti-depressant, anti-anxiety, uplifting, antispasmodic, anti-inflammatory, aphrodisiac, an aid to deeper sleep, and a benefit to the skin and hair care.

Suggested Uses: Clary sage should not be used during pregnancy, but it can be very useful during labor. It is believed to induce and strengthen contractions and reduce stress and tensions. For treatment of premenstrual symptoms, blend 3 to 6 drops of clary sage with 1 to 2 drops of rose otto and 3 to 5 drops of lavender and add to a tub full of warm bathwater.

JASMINE ABSOLUTE (Jasminum officinale or Jasmine grandiflorum)
Nature: Jasmine, sweet jasmine is one scent everyone loves. It is deep, sweet, floral, and rich. Real jasmine, like rose, cannot be compared to the imitation fragrances that fill shop shelves. I recall attending a birth where the room was redolent of jasmine from a massage oil the mother was using while walking before birth. I made it for her bless-away gift: a little something to wish mother and child good luck. (See more about bless aways on page 127.) Jasmine has been known to help instill self-confidence, and when giving birth we need all the confidence we can get!

Benefits: Believed to be antidepressant, warming, antianxiety, beneficial to the skin and scalp, aphrodisiac, emotionally balancing, soothing, warming, antiseptic, expectorant, and sedative. Jasmine is uplifting and seems to enhance confidence. Jasmine equally benefits men and women.

SUGGESTED ESSENTIAL OILS FOR THE BATH

Following is a list of some of the most commonly used essential oils, along with their benefits. The whole fresh or dried herb or fruit (fresh slices of lemons work wonders) can also be used in the bath.

- ◆ Bergamot: to balance
- ◆ Eucalyptus: to clear and open
- ◆ Frankincense: to bless and repair
- ◆ Lavender: to unwind
- ◆ Lemon: to brighten and refresh
- ◆ Roman Chamomile: to relax
- ◆ Rose: to soothe the soul
- ◆ Rosemary: to stimulate or remember
- ◆ Sandalwood: to soothe the spirit

For depression, wear jasmine as a personal essence to envelope you throughout the day in a fragrance that has been cherished for centuries by many cultures. Just breathing in jasmine is believed to benefit the respiratory system. Added to skin-care products and hair oils, it soothes and moisturizes.

Blend jasmine with patchouli, rose, sandalwood, and ylang-ylang to bring out the sensuality often repressed due to stress, anxiety, or depression.

Suggested Uses: Jasmine is the oil of choice to massage a mother about to give birth, but is too stimulating to be used in early pregnancy. Jasmine helps lift depression, which can be a problem after giving birth. What a wonderful shower gift for an expectant mother, a bottle of jasmine massage oil. Use a very diluted blend and a small amount at a time. It can be costly, but like rose, well worth the expense.

I dilute jasmine in jojoba oil; this blend keeps longer than one in sweet almond oil. Only a very small amount of jasmine is ever needed. Do not be tempted to use more for a greater effect. This may actually have an opposite result. Less is best; besides, the cost of good, true, jasmine will limit its use for most of us.

LAVENDER (*Lavandula officinalis*)

Nature: Lavender's classic floral/herbal scent has been treasured for centuries as a washing herb, and has freshened many a bed linen. Its name evolved from the Latin *lavare,* which means "to wash."

Benefits: Lavender essential oil has been found effective in cases of stress, insomnia, acne, infection, anxiety, depression, headaches, skin irritations (burns, eczema), and fatigue.

Suggested Uses: Lavender is an oil that I count on for small scrapes and insect stings. It is one of the few oils that I feel safe using "neat," or undiluted on my skin. It is a favorite when a blemish pops up at just the wrong time. I simply put a drop on a cotton swab and apply it to the spot. It is very useful in skin care because of its cytophylactic, or cell-protecting and regenerating properties.

ROSE (*Rosa gallica, Rosa damascena, Rosa centifolia*)

Nature: Once you have inhaled the heavenly scent of rose otto or absolute, you will never again accept an imitation rose fragrance!

Benefits: Rose oil has been found effective in cases of depression, insomnia, impotence, skin care, nervous tension, feminine complaints, grief, sadness, and low self-esteem.

Use: Rosewater has been employed as a skin-care agent for centuries. Rose absolute is obtained when roses are extracted through the enfluerage method. This reddish liquid is just the remedy for emotional imbalances, reminding us to love ourselves. I add rose otto to a night facial oil as an occasional luxurious ritual. Treat yourself or someone you love to a bottle of rose absolute or otto. Just a little dab can have a great effect on body, mind, and spirit.

Carrier or Base Oils

Carrier or base oils are the substances that pure essential oils are diluted into for various preparations, including bath, body, facial, and massage products. Use only high-quality carrier oils to blend your products and mix only as much as you can use quickly, to prevent oxidation. The scent of rancid carrier oil is not pleasant and will cling to towels, sheets, and clothing.

Bases like sweet almond, grapeseed, apricot kernel, avocado, and jojoba are oily to the touch. Others include cream and gel bases. Some people prefer good cream or lotion bases as opposed to oily ones. I use all of them, depending on the type of skin care or treatment I'm making.

When selecting a base, make sure it is of as high a quality as your pure essential oils. There is no sense in putting fine oils in a synthetic or mineral oil base.

Most essential oil companies carry a variety of bases, but you may choose to experiment with making your own. Aloe vera gel can be used when a cream or oil base isn't appropriate. Here are some of the carriers you may want to have on hand to experiment with.

SWEET ALMOND OIL
Nature: Great base for massage, bath, body, and skin care products. Sweet almond oil is scentless and nourishing to the skin.
Benefits: Sweet almond oil relieves dry skin and may be used by itself, unscented, just to condition the skin. I like to apply it after a shower to my still-damp skin. It emulsifies with the water and blends in nicely. The addition of pure essential oils adds to an individual's skin care regimen. I also use this along with jojoba oil for a hair oil treatment.

JOJOBA OIL
Nature: This liquid wax will solidify when allowed to get too cool. It is an excellent base for personal essences because it doesn't "go off" or become rancid as quickly as some of the others will. I use it to extend costly oils like rose, jasmine, sandalwood, and linden. I always list this dilution on my products so my clients know when a particular oil has been cut. It is a good avenue to allow people to experience an oil at a lesser cost than if they bought it undiluted. A 10 percent dilution works well.
Benefits: Jojoba is nourishing to the skin and hair. I use one-third part jojoba oil in hair oils.

GRAPESEED OIL

Nature: This oily base is much lighter to the touch than most others. I like it to massage the back because my hands seem to glide over a larger area easier. It is less viscous than other bases. One year I obtained some fresh from a winery. It was the best I had ever used. Its green hue can be detected even in amber bottles. I use this alone or combined with sweet almond for massage.

APRICOT KERNEL OIL

Nature: Full of vitamins and minerals, this oily base is good for skin-care products for all types of skin. It is especially useful on sensitive and aging skin. I refer to this as "mature skin." (At Herbal Endeavours Ltd., we consider any skin more than 20 years old to be mature.)

AVOCADO OIL

Nature: This is nice as 10 percent of a facial oil. It is beneficial to all skins and contains vitamins and fatty acids.

WHEAT GERM OIL

Nature: Also good to the skin, this yellow oil when added in a 10 percent ratio to a skin-care product will help extend its shelf life and benefit the skin with its high vitamin, mineral, and protein content.

OTHER BASES

Essential oils may also be added to already existing products such as shampoos, conditioners, skin lotions, dish soap, cleaning bases, water for household sprays, alcohol for perfumes, sea salt, and powder bases.

LEARNING TO USE ESSENTIAL OILS

Pick up a few really good books on herbs and beauty to give you some ideas about what you'd like to try. The best way to learn is to get in there and try by blending a little bit at a time. Abide by all cautions and let your nose, knowledge, and intuition be your guides. Start with very small amounts of oils — only 1 or 2 drops per application — and see what works best for you.

Keep a pencil and pad of paper available to record you experiments, successes, and failures.

Always make sure that your products are well mixed and shaken to keep the pure essential oils evenly distributed in them. Make up small batches, fresh. These products aren't meant to have a long shelf life; there aren't any or only a small amount of natural preservatives in them. Be sure to label what you have added and the date.

Equipment for Working with Essential Oils

Dark glass bottles. You'll need clean, dark glass bottles of varying sizes to store your mixtures; bottles that hold 1 dram (4 ml) to 8 ounces are ideal. Well-washed old vitamin and tincture bottles work well. Now is the opportunity to fill those pretty perfume bottles and decorative jars you've been wondering how to use. Filled with some of your products, they'll make lovely gifts.

Spray bottles. Have a supply in various sizes, 4 to 16 ounces. These come in handy for everything to spritzing rosewater upon your face to clearing the air where your pets play. These spray bottles, when well shaken, will enable you to propel pure essential oils and water over the body, home, or vehicle. Make sure these spray bottles are scrupulously clean and do not contain the residue of any toxic substance. I often buy these new for healing and reuse ones for home cleaning or car care.

Glass eyedroppers. The rubber tops of these will eventually break down from contact with the pure essential oils. Try to collect pure essential oils with dropper tops to avoid this, and try to keep the oil off the rubber part of the dropper.

Glass beakers and glass mixing rods. These are to mix blends in and to bottle with later. Your oil blend pours evenly out of these. I have filled many bottles this way. You may also just mix in the bottle you intend to keep the blend in and shake it gently. Try to keep bottles full to prevent too much oxidation of the blended oils.

Labels. Label everything with the ingredients, date, and use. Creative labels will enhance an essential oil collection. The label is a very important part of a perfume. It must convey in print and picture what the perfumer wants you to imagine its scent is like. It is almost impossible to imagine a never-before-experienced scent, so this label must be effective to pique your interest. Why do you think so much is now spent on the bottle and packaging of a perfume and so much less on contents? (I wouldn't mind a plain, amber bottle that is filled with jasmine absolute at all!)

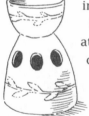

Diffuser. This electric device blends air and pure essential oils without heating them. It sprays a fine mist out into a room. I have seen and tried many prototypes of these little machines. Many I tried actually were damaged by the undiluted oils. The oils marred the plastic surfaces, and the tubing had to be replaced. Use caution in choosing a place to set them. I know people who swear by these diffusers and wouldn't be without one. They can be expensive to buy and operate, depending on the pure essential oils you use. You also can put one on a timer. I once played around with making an aromatic alarm clock of rosemary and lemon. It was fun, although I am quite time oriented and rarely need or use an alarm clock. Not everyone is so lucky, though, and some people have a difficult time being awakened in the morning. What a lovely way to start the day!

Simmer pot. It seems everyone has received one of these at some point in their lives to simmer potpourri. Some are candle heated and some are electric. I fill them with water and add the desired essential oils to the water. Keep an eye on the water level. These work well outside to drive away

CAUTION ON USING HEAT SOURCES

Keep a keen eye on any heat source you employ to release the scent of your essential oils. Candles, simmer pots, and light bulb rings can catch fire if not properly attended. Forgo these methods if you are ill or sleepy. On these occasions a diffuser on a timer will serve you much better. Oils on cotton or a small cloth can work well then, too.

unwanted bugs and in the house when someone has been ill. I use one when I have a head cold or chest congestion so I can inhale the vapors of the pure essential oils.

Aroma lamp. These are like simmer pots but without the water. Pure essential oils are added directly to a warming area and diffuse. These lamps may be very elaborate in their design. Again, these are candle or electrically heated and must be used with caution.

Aroma jewelry. This is becoming quite popular. I have collected aroma jewelry for more than ten years. I have several necklaces that contain a compartment for pure essential oils to be added. I also own a pair of earrings with a place to add a few drops of oil. My favorite is a gift I cherish. It is called a posy pin. It's a small glass vase on a stickpin. I fill the pin with water and place small flowers and herbs in it. This little treasure keeps my flowers fresh all day long and when placed on my lapel I can enjoy their scent while I work. Sometimes I place it on a hat, also. I love to fill it with Johnny-jump-up, lily-of-the-valley, miniature roses, spearmint, violets, thyme, lavender, chamomile flowers, and soapwort.

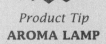

Product Tip
AROMA LAMP

You can obtain a lovely electric aroma lamp from Star Power Essentials (see resource list). This is a ceramic diffuser that operates silently on a 25-watt bulb. It comes with extra ceramic basins so you can change the essential oil easily.

Storing Essential Oils

Store essential oils well away from heat, light, and air in well-sealed, full, dark-glass, dropper-top bottles with proper labeling. They should be stored well away from children and homeopathic remedies.

Buy small amounts whenever possible. Air in unfilled bottles can help to impair pure essential oils. Try to keep your bottles cool, dark, and well filled. Transfer oils to a smaller bottle if you do not need them for a while.

Preparing Dilutions and Solutions

The common dilution is 1 to 3 drops essential oil to 100 drops carrier. Approximately 1 drop essential to 2 mls carrier oil = 2½ percent solution. A 1 percent solution is used for facial oils and for children over the age of two. Use with babies should be researched thoroughly before implementing. Up to 3 percent is common for massage therapy and body oils for older children (ages 7–14) and adults. Always use an eyedropper or dropper-top bottle to dispense.

Dilution Guidelines

Less is Best. Always opt on the side of caution when using pure essential oils. Start out with a mere ½ percent solution, especially when using on children, elderly, or those with sensitive skin or face.

For babies up to 3 months old, keep the application of lotions, powder, creams, and such to a bare minimum. The acceptable concentration depends on a variety of factors: age, size of the area to be massaged, how oils are being employed, and strengh and intensity of specific oil(s) being used. Always obtain the highest quality, most pure essential oils you can. Here are a few basic dilution formulas:

Dilution Solution	Formula
½ percent	3 drops essential oil to 30 ml (2 tablespoons) carrier oil or base
1 percent	3 drops essential oil to 15 ml (1 tablespoon) carrier oil or base
2 percent	6 drops essential oil to 15 ml (1 tablespoon) carrier oil or base
3 percent	9 drops essential oil to 15 ml (1 tablespoon) carrier oil or base

HOMEOPATHY

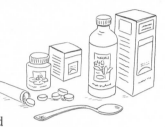

The practice of homeopathy goes way back in history. Modern homeopathy is almost 200 years old. It originated in Europe, where it is still practiced by a large percentage of doctors and the general population. Dr. Samuel Hahnemann is credited with being the founder of homeopathy. It was once popular here in the United States, fell out of favor, and now is on a tremendous rebound.

Homeopathic remedies are subtle, but care with their use must be observed. I can't imagine life with children and no homeopathics. They are designated as over-the-counter remedies, and are now available in many chain pharmacies.

What Is a Homeopathic Remedy?

From the Greek *homios,* meaning "similar," and *pathos,* meaning "disorder," the concept homeopathy is that "like treats like." These remedies are similar in action to vaccines and allergy shots, which are a minute amount of a substance used to stimulate a reaction in the body that is like the substance used, or to build immunity to it. Remedies are made from botanical, mineral, and animal sources. They are easy to use, and normally pretty agreeable to the children who need to employ their powers. They are reported to have very few side effects. Not habit-forming and available in most health food shops and by mail order, Mother Nature's little helpers are worth investigating.

These traditional healers enable us to aid our families on a deeper level because homeopathy treats the person as a whole, and is based on symptomatologies using recognized remedies for alleviation. A minute dose of a substance that can cause a similar reaction to the condition you are working to heal enables the person's body to deal better naturally to heal itself by stimulating it on its own. This is referred to as the defensive-reactive process. The remedy produces similar mental and physical symptoms as the condition. Like heals like. There are lovely home-use homeopathy books available today, many with color pictures and easy-to-read descriptions of various remedies (see reading list). There are even computer programs and CD-roms that teach you how to work with homeopathic remedies.

Always consult a homeopathic physician for other than simple minor discomforts or ailments. Deeper-seated problems and complaints require professional observation and evaluation.

How Are Remedies Used?

Homeopathic remedies come in various potencies and forms, but usually as a small white pellet or tablet. They are most often

Product Tips
HOMEOPATHY

Homeopathic Education Services of Berkeley, CA (see resource list) offers an excellent catalog and information packet. This is another of my "where were you when my kids were small?" companies. It offers one-stop shopping for quality books and remedies. Titles in the catalog include *Homeopathic Medicines for Pregnancy and Childbirth* by Richard Moskowitz, M.D.; *Homeopathy for Pregnancy, Birth, and First Year* by Miranda Castro, RSHom.; *Homeopathy for Birthing* by Jana Willen Jansen; *Homeopathic Medicine for Children and Infants* by Dana Ullman, MPH; and many family-oriented titles. Products offered include the kit that I refer to as my healing blue and white box, which they call Le Kit. It contains 36 medicines of varying potencies and four external applications. A perfect kit to start out with is their Beginners Kit, or The Children's Kit. The Children's Kit contains some of the most common remedies in thirty X for pediatric problems. Included are aconitum, arnica, belladonna, and chamomilla. Articles, posters, slides, software, and cassette tapes are also available.

in a lactose base. Sometimes they are in a liquid form. These are all usually held under the tongue and allowed to melt.

Homeopathic remedies are normally available in health food stores. Although using them is very simple, there are a few precautions that need to be followed. Do not use homeopathic remedies at the same time you are using mint or any product containing camphor (like Vicks VapoRub) or liniments, as these may interfere with them. Also, remember to discontinue use once the symptoms improve or clear up.

COMMON HOMEOPATHIC REMEDIES AND THEIR TRADITIONAL USES

There are some basic homeopathic remedies that I have always found useful in my household, belladonna, chamomilla, arnica, apis, Rhus toxicodendron, and calendula to name a few. Nature's Products, a great little herb shop in Detroit from which I have purchased herbs, homeopathic remedies, pure essential oils, vitamin supplements, and books for more than ten years, has been a great resource. I have called owner Gary Wanttaja many times to ask which herbs and remedies he has found successful in his own life and in those of the community he serves. However, I am always responsible to know what I want to use as much because I know neither he nor anyone else can really prescribe for people. Know what you want when you order herbs and homeopathic remedies. Take some time, if possible, to get to know these natural allies. You never know when you will need them, when it's up to you to soothe a family member, or perhaps yourself.

CAUTION

Before you embark on a homeopathic course of treatment, be sure to refer to a more in-depth book on homeopathy (see reading list). Any child who does not respond to a homeopathic remedy or other home care within five or six hours should receive prompt medical attention.

How They Are Administered

Homeopathic remedies usually come in an easy-to-administer small white pellet that is dissolved under the tongue. The pellet is placed under the tongue directly from the plastic insert cap (on a tube) or the cap of a small bottle. It is commonly believed that the pellets should not be touched. However, for children I think just getting it in their mouth, and not worrying about it being under the tongue, is sufficient. A common dosage of a homeopathic remedy is 4 to 6 pellets. Some remedies also come in a liquid dose dropper-top bottle. Before taking anything, be sure to check the directions from the specific supplier. Taking a class or having a professional consultation from a practicing homeopathic physician can help you get started.

Gary Wanttaja generously shared a list of his favorite homeopathic remedies, combined here with some of mine.

ACONITE
Use: Useful at first onset of symptoms for fever, colds, flu, with restlessness and anxiety, usually brought on by sudden exposure to cold, dry weather.

APIS
Nature: Apis is actually crushed bee on a pellet. I always carry it in my pocket when I am gardening or visiting gardens.
Use: Treat bee stings and hives. Apis was helpful to me one summer day when I was planting lavender for a client and a bee thought it would be a lovely time to take a walk up inside my sunglasses. My reaction was just that, a reaction, and not a very calm one. Being excitable too, Mr. Bee promptly stung me between my eye and my nose — no fun! I took a dose of Apis and went to a nearby restaurant for a small glass of ice and a napkin to hold it in to apply to my swollen face. In about ten minutes the sting began to subside even without the ice and by the time I arrived home, about two hours later, only a small red puncture wound and slight swelling were left. I carried Apis around so much that I wore the name off the bottle. I also employed it once when a hornet decided to take a snooze under the rim of one of my large flowerpots of rose geranium. When I picked up the pot to move it, I disturbed him and he gave me a wake-up call! Ouch! Apis! Ice!

ARNICA
Nature: Arnica is mountain daisy. Blessed Arnica! Where would we be without Arnica? I carry this remedy everywhere I go.

Use: Very useful for common bumps, bruises, and simple injuries, reducing swelling and trauma. The gel has soothed tired feet from climbing castle stairs in England, and in pellet form eased the pain of a wisdom tooth coming in for a young adult. It was a godsend for bumped and bruised little boo-boos. I have employed Arnica for sore, overworked muscles and for sore tissue when I came too close to various objects and sustained a bump or bruise. I love Arnica in gel form, as a pellet, in a variety of dosages depending on the condition. Arnica has helped me deal with Luggage Shoulders and Garden Back, two common ailments, in the form of a massage oil from Weleda Products in Spring Valley, New York (see page 148). For little ones, Arnica Spray works on those boo-boos that are just too sore to touch.

Arnica should not be used on open or broken skin. Arnica isn't commonly used in its herb form, and should only be employed as a homeopathic remedy in the form of gels, pellets, oils, and sprays.

ARSENICUM ALBUM
Use: Helpful for stomach flu when accompanied by restlessness, anxiety, excessive thirst, and chills.

BELLADONNA
Nature: Nightshade. This herb is poisonous in all other forms. It can also cause excessive vomiting.

Use: Fever; chicken pox; common colds; or earache with symptoms of flushed face, dry mouth, and glassy eyes with quick onset of symptoms. Homeopathically it has aided my daughter with sudden hot fevers. I do not give medication to stop a fever unless absolutely necessary. I watch her and usually give her belladonna or chamomilla. Fevers in new borns and small or young infants should be evaluated by a physician since meningitis is a possibility.

Belladonna is for her hot red cheeks, fever, and the suddenness with which her symptoms always arise. Whether she has an infection or a cold, the sudden high fever is her way of showing it. Belladonna seems to help her aching, throbbing head, sore throat, sore ears, and sensitivity to noise, light, and strong odors. My daughter is 16 and we still use these basic remedies regularly. I trust that I am helping her make choices in her healthcare practices as an adult. Also, she hates to swallow pills or medicines the color of bubblegum. She prefers the pleasant-tasting, easy-to-dissolve-under-the tongue pellets. Her quick, often amazing recoveries have shown us the power of homeopathic remedies.

CALCAREA CARBONICA
Use: Earache, common cold, colic, child generally has many fears and tends to be chilly.

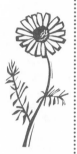

CHAMOMILLA
Nature: From the herb chamomile, which has a centuries-old reputation for calming and soothing mankind. This was my cranky-kid godsend.
Use: Soothes earache, colic, teething, especially with irritable, restless disposition. I valued it during colic, teething, earaches, stressful times; for my daughter and me, it would bring relief on days when we were both too short of patience to be nice. Temper tantrums were a bit shorter lived when this or Rescue Remedy was employed early on. When I was nursing, I took them and nursed her if she wasn't feeling well or after I had a bad day. Always consult proper medical supervision when nursing before using any drugs, herbs, pure essential oils, or natural remedies. HyLands offers a line of children's remedies with chamomilla in some of them. These include: Colic Tablets, Calms Forte, Calms, and Teething Tablets (available from P & S Laboratories, a division of Standard Homeopathic Company in Los Angeles, California, see source list).

EUPATORIUM PERFOLIATUM
Use: Flu with characteristic achy bones and chills.

GELSEMIUM
Use: Flu with achiness and child is drowsy, droopy, chilly, and not thirsty.

MERCURIUS
Use: Sore throat, often with swollen glands, colds with green-ish discharge that can spread to ears or throat.

NATRUM MURIATICUM

Use: Colds with a clear or thick white discharge; child desires to be left alone and rejects sympathy.

PULSATILLA

Use: Colds with a yellow-green discharge and child is moody, weepy, clingy, and seeks comfort and sympathy.

RHUS TOXICODENDRON/POISON IVY

Nature: That's right, poison ivy. Hard to believe anyone in his right mind would give a child poison anything! This is where the infinitesimal dose comes in. As in all homeopathic remedies, these are very diluted in strength or potentized. Samuel Hahnemann, homeopathy's father, said, "In order to bring about prompt, gentle, and lasting improvement, you most often need to use infinitesimal doses." Because they are so weak, they no longer act upon us like their namesakes. They actually stimulate us naturally to respond.

Use: Flu with achiness, dry cough, restlessness, child tosses and turns and craves cold drinks. Chicken pox. Poison ivy.

Rhus tox, as I refer to it, is just the one when I have a rash after working in the gardens. I sometimes come across an unknown plant in a handful of weeding and have a reaction. Little fluid-filled red spots are usually short lived after Rhus Tox (same with poison ivy or oak). The last time I encountered poison ivy it was lovingly transported to me upon the back of my beloved kitty Rosemary, who rubbed against my legs after she encountered the plant. So keep this in mind with children. You don't have to be in the middle of a woods to come in contact; only the family pet does.

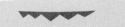

A WORD OF WARNING

Always place all healing remedies in locked or inaccessible containers. Don't store your pure essential oils and herbs along with your homeopathic remedies. Store them separately, away from one another. Being stored together can adversely affect the potency.

This remedy has helped me with flu-like symptoms of fever, body aches, and stiffness of joints. I have found this effective in hives, cold sores, eczema, and chicken pox.

SULPHUR

Use: Measles, sore throat, impetigo, or if child is uncharacteristically warm even when well.

BACH FLOWER REMEDIES

After giving up a conventional medical practice in the early 1930's, Dr. Edward Bach wandered the countryside of England searching for remedies for the emotional changes that he believed were at the root of our physical ills. In his book, *Health Thyself and Free Thyself,* Bach outlined his Twelve Healers. He eventually revealed thirty-eight remedies he worked with. These are simply flower-charged waters that are often preserved in brandy. Often confused with essential oils, these remedies are actually homeopathic-like in nature. They are gentle, easy-to-use, safe, and have been found highly effective to treat many symptoms. The Bach Flower Remedies are administered in a glass of water or by placing directly under the tongue and allowing to dissolve.

Bach Rescue Remedy

One of the most well-known Bach Flower Remedies, Rescue Remedy, is actually a blend of five ingredients: Star of Bethlehem (to neutralize the mental or physical effects of shock or grievous disappointment); Rock Rose (to treat terror, panic, or extreme fright as a result of an accident or nightmare); Impatience (for stress, irritability, impatience, or mental tension); Cherry Plum (for desperation, fear of doing something out of control, or losing your mind); and Clematis (to treat inattention, preoccupation, lack of concentration, or the spacey feeling that often accompanies stressful situations). Just four drops of Rescue Remedy in a glass of water helps many people ease tensions.

For parents, a working knowledge of Bach Flower Remedies can offer a bit of sanity and peace in times of upheaval. They are safe, inexpensive, and easy to use.

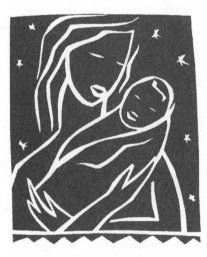

Caring for Yourself
During Pregnancy,
Childbirth, and
Lactation

CHAPTER

Pregnancy and childbirth are experiences that stay firmly with us throughout a lifetime, or shall I say lifetimes — yours and your child's. These experiences are recalled and related many times over in the course of a parent-child relationship and are worth putting in the effort to explore the very best options available during these experiences, for both you and your child.

Pregnancy is a time when everything is changing very rapidly, including your physical being, your emotional life (both internally and with your partner, friends, and other supportive members of your community), and your life perspective. It is a time to reach out and acquire the very best resources nature has to offer. These are very special days in the endless cycle we call life, yet often we spend more time researching the options for a new car or interest rates on a new house than we do the options for a natural and healthy pregnancy, childbirth, lactation, and child care. Yes these rhythms are natural, but mother nature has some tired and true clues for you towards the best beginnings.

When considering pregnancy, you must first take your general health into account. If you're planning to conceive, take a look at your diet and lifestyle, including over-the-counter medications and natural remedies you may use, and the stress level in your life.

PREPARING FOR CONCEPTION

Nature doesn't always give you the opportunity to know in advance when you'll conceive, so it's wise to try your best to maintain a healthy lifestyle if you're a woman of childbearing years (as it is for women of all ages). The best way to a healthy baby is through a healthy mother and father. Today is always a great day to start living better. When you have a little one on the way, you will need all of the strength and energy that a healthier lifestyle will afford you. This will be a time of profound change, and they will be there for a long time to come.

Importance of Relaxation

Infertility has plagued many couples, and opting for better health and learning how to relax a bit can sometimes go a long way toward helping to conceive. I don't mean to make light of infertility problems; you should search out competent help. However, relaxation is an important ingredient of conception. I have friends who were so uptight about having a baby that they completely stressed themselves to the point that they were almost ill. Conflict, blame, grief, anticipation, and disappointment all fill the air.

Bach Rescue Remedy (a homeopathic remedy) is useful in easing states of high stress and anxiety and restoring balance. Rescue Remedy is administered by combining 4 drops with a small glass of water and sipping slowly, or by putting 4 drops directly under the tongue. I carry a bottle of this remedy in a pocket of my purse and have indeed found it a godsend in high-stress situations. It is very helpful at easing shock, grief, and

BEWARE OF HOUSEHOLD PRODUCTS

Just as it's important to be careful about using essential oils during pregnancy, it's equally wise to be aware of the other potent materials you're exposed to during pregnancy. Read labels! Know what you're using. Obtain a book that explains the ingredients in common household products.

I became acutely aware of this dilemma when expecting my daughter. While I carefully watched my diet and lifestyle to ensure a healthy pregnancy, I realized that the prepackaged, chemically treated ingredients in my shampoo, conditioner, body lotion, styling products, and perfumes presented just as much danger as did the other factors I was seeking to control. This was the inspiration I needed to delve deeper into the art of creating my own health- and beauty-care products at home. This became my business, but it was a necessity first. I didn't want to try so hard to keep healthy throughout the pregnancy and then fill my child's life with drugs if she were ill or with chemical-laden baby products.

everyday emotional growing pains. Pure essential oils, our aromatic allies, can also contribute to the relief of stress when used in baths, massage, inhalations, and personal perfumes.

PREGNANCY

The body undergoes tremendous changes throughout pregnancy and birth. It changes from one life to two and rides an ebb and flow of hormone fluctuations. The skin is usually stretched to capacity, and the hair and nails may either

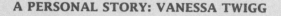

A PERSONAL STORY: VANESSA TWIGG

I had the pleasure of meeting aromatherapist Vanessa Twigg during a recent visit to England. Vanessa completed her general nursing training in 1985 and became a mental health nurse in 1989. She currently is studying aromatology at the International College of Aromatherapy and will receive her diploma in nursing as part of the B.A. in medical science with Sheffield University Hospital. She plans to open an aromatherapy school.

Vanessa was kind enough to share the profile of her pregnancies. Here she describes her aromatic experiences.

"While pregnant with my first child I had not long been qualified in aromatherapy. I sadly chose not to use aromatherapy during my pregnancy. I had taught that no oil is 100 percent safe to use during pregnancy, only tangerine. Being pregnant in the summer, and having both a hot summer and a skin that was sensitive during this time, I was worried that the discoloration on my body and face would be worse, due to the mild risk of photosensitization of the citrus oils.

"I was nauseous all the way through, lost 20 pounds, was anemic, and although I wanted to have a home delivery, I felt obliged to go into hospital due to outside pressures. I had a particularly difficult birth due to the position of the baby, had to have pethidine and morphine, which caused hallucinations, and which also caused the baby to also be drugged, a slow feeder, and slightly hypothermic — issues that were not too serious, but as a new mother knows, there is enough anxiety without adding more."

When her daughter was four months old, Vanessa found herself pregnant with her second child. "I made my mind up there and then that things would be different this time. I had been offered a job working within a natural health center, and didn't want to turn this opportunity down or have to stop working. I also improve or worsen according to an individual's state of health and diet. I encourage you to work very closely with a doctor, nurse/midwife, naturopathic physician, and/or nutritionist to ensure your child nature's best beginning.

Using Pure Essential Oils

The use of pure essential oils during pregnancy and childbirth has sparked much controversy. I have heard a variety of recommendations, from using some oils throughout pregnancy to

didn't want to go through the sickness as before. I booked in with my homeopath and started to drink fennel tea and use fennel hydrosol to prevent nausea. I am thankful that I was not sick once. I drank recommended iron seaweed drink, which helped to naturally keep my iron levels up. Although I was apparently still anemic from the first child, I never felt tired or ill. I planned to have my baby at home with the help of a midwife (this was, in fact, kept a secret from everyone, even my husband, until I had the baby, so as to avoid the pressure of a hospital admission). I learned exercises to help encourage the baby to be in the correct position.

"I continued to work as a therapist until I was too big to massage, as my 'lump' prevented me from getting near to a couch. I only had six weeks off. I also continued to use all my aromatherapy oils, and gave myself massage and aromatic baths weekly.

"I continued to see the homeopath monthly, which helped immensely, not only with the pregnancy, but also with my moods due to hormone changes.

I was given a little supply of homeopathic remedies to take home for labor. With the help of both aromatherapy and homeopathy over the phone during labor, I was able to have a very nice, quick, easy home birth. I never thought that I would say this, but I thoroughly enjoyed the experience. My son was born healthy at 8:45 P.M., and slept happily until 7:00 A.M. the next day. This meant that I could get my rest. The next day I felt the happiest and healthiest of my life, full of energy and enthusiasm.

"I do not know how, if at all, different things would have been if I had not used aromatherapy and homeopathy. I make no claims, but I feel that it made a remarkable difference to me, my pregnancy, the birth, and both my and my baby's health. If I was to find myself pregnant again, then I know which route I would take without hesitation."

using them only in the last trimester, to avoiding them altogether. I maintain a middle ground, recommending the use of only a few select oils, usually in high dilution. I try always to err on the side of caution.

Use caution. If you are newly pregnant or trying to conceive, a light hand with pure essential oils is the best route. Few adverse effects have actually been reported to me. However, you must be sensitive, aware of what the oils are doing. If you are at high risk for any complications in pregnancy, or have a history of miscarriage, pure essential oils must be considered only with the advice of a doctor, nurse/midwife, qualified aromatologist, aromatherapist, medical herbalist, or naturopathic doctor.

First and foremost, get an honest evaluation of your present health. The body undergoes profound changes during the time it takes to produce a child. Hormonal changes cause a variety of bodily changes — not all of them to our liking.

Pregnancy is a natural process, and with proper medical advice pure essential oils can be a part of this wondrous time. There is one caution I cannot stress enough about essential oils: Do not underestimate their power. These oils are highly concentrated and extremely potent. They are very different from homeopathic remedies and from Bach Flower Remedies, which are already greatly diluted when they come into your hands. If working with essential oils is new for you, be particularly careful.

I say all this not to scare you, but to encourage you to use caution in making or buying fine natural products. (See page 26 for more detailed information on working with essential oils.) I believe it is the improper choice of oil, lack of respect for proper dilution, and the incorrect method of application, not the actual pure essential oils themselves, that bring about problems.

Different oils for different purposes. Pure essential oils can be helpful allies in soothing some of the common discomforts associated with pregnancy, including nausea, mood swings, backache, problem skin, aching feet, emotional stress, fatigue, insomnia, and muscle tension. Some oils are best used in one way, while others are best administered in another way. For instance, 1 or 2 drops of Roman chamomile added to a foot bath or a compress makes a great relaxant for someone in the late second to third trimester of pregnancy. Peppermint is another oil that can be used in this fashion during the late second to third trimester to soothe and cool the body. Other oils, such as frankincense, are best employed as an inhalation in a simmer pot to treat a pregnant woman's chest congestion during the last two trimesters. Still other pure essential oils lend themselves well to the bath, a massage oil, or bath salts. These include lavender and rose geranium, which can both be used in low-percentage dilutions during the second two trimesters.

Lemon, bergamot, and most other citrus oils are phototoxic; that is, they react when they are exposed to light. Avoid these or use them with caution if you are going to be outside or exposed to strong sunlight. Be sure to check on the specific guidelines for each oil.

Learn as much as you can. Knowledge is the key to all things, natural and otherwise. When in doubt, check it out. I have found that doing as much research on your own as possible greatly lessens the chances of misusing any natural remedies. Ask questions until you feel you have the answers you need to make a safe, confident decision as to the importance pure essential oils will have in your life and that of your family. Make phone calls, write letters, go to classes, visit herb shops and aromatherapy stores, and ask the voice of experience whenever possible.

A mountain of information on pure essential oils is being generated every day. As people learn and grow, they are often eager to share their stories. Be sure to use your local library as

---

Product Tip
MOTHER'S ULTIMATE BELLY OIL

While browsing on the internet, I discovered a company's web page at http://www.eden.com advertising their product Mother's Ultimate Belly Oil. This is a rich blend of base oils such as sweet almond oil, wheat germ oil, Borage seed oil, carrot seed oil, and jojoba oil combined with pure essential oils of lavender, tangerine, neroli, rose, and rose geranium. This informative page goes on to advise applying this blend twice a day to any area that is taut, including hips, stomach, breasts, thighs, and buttocks. Ahhhhhhhh! The page also includes some information on nutrition, advice for avoiding stretch marks, and guidance on alternative birthing practices.

well as a personal home computer to help you in your quest to learn more about alternative options during pregnancy. There are many conversations and information-sharing sessions taking place on the internet.

Massage Techniques

Avoid any essential oil massage during the first three months of pregnancy. Energy work or just light massage application of plain carrier oils may be all that is needed during this early stage of pregnancy. Energy work includes techniques such as reiki, polarity, or meditation which address the energy or aura surrounding the body more than the physical body itself. While full body massage (*without* essential oils) is not necessarily contraindicated in the first trimester, it is not advised for women with varicose veins in pregnancy because of the risk of DVM/ deep vein thrombosis.

When a body massage is not advisable, hand and foot massage is an effective way of relaxing the body and releasing tension. A neck and shoulder massage is another great way to unwind and relax. Be sure to take care of yourself by requesting these treatments from a loved one, or a massage therapist, when stress begins to creep in. A foot bath will also provide great relief after a long day or add comfort to a sleepless night.

COMMUNICATING BEFORE BIRTH

The feelings you and your mate have from conception are transmitted to your baby. The more positive you can make the experience, the better start you'll have on a strong relationship with your child. Meditation, telepathic communication, and visualization are powerful tools with which to communicate with your child before birth. The sound of your voice is also very important to your child in utero. Talk to your baby from the time it is conceived. Favorite music can also be a powerful way to share and communicate with your child before birth. I played a music box to Christina the whole time I was expecting and she seemed to recognize its music after she was born.

Neck and Shoulder Massage. The muscles of the head and neck can become stiff with the stress and strain of everyday life. A head, neck, backbone, and shoulder massage can be a great stress reliever and help prevent the stress from creeping deeper into your muscles.

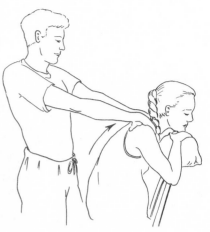

Following are some neck and shoulder massage oil recipes especially for pregnant women. *Note:* When I say ONE drop of oil I literally mean ONE drop (especially in regards to rosemary and peppermint oils). Some people might say these recipes are on the light side, but I believe in always erring on the side of caution. When developing your own formulas, be sure to check which oils should not be used in early pregnancy (see page 21). Don't worry about getting the oil in your hair, it will serve as a conditioning treatment.

COMBINATION #1
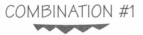

1 tablespoon base oil or lotion
1 drop Roman chamomile essential oil
1 drop lavender essential oil

COMBINATION #2
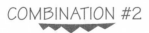

1 tablespoon base oil or lotion
1 drop neroli essential oil
1 drop lavender essential oil

COMBINATION #3
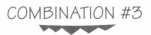

1 tablespoon base oil or lotion
1 drop ylang-ylang essential oil
1 drop patchouli essential oil

COMBINATION #4

For a quick pick-me-up when you must carry on with your day try the following:

> 1 tablespoon base oil or lotion
> 1 drop rosemary essential oil
> 1 drop lemon essential oil
> **OR**
> 1 tablespoon base oil or lotion
> 1 drop peppermint essential oil
> 1 drop rose geranium essential oil

Body massage. After three months of pregnancy or when advised by your attending physician, midwife, or aromatherapist, abdominal massage can help you through your pregnancy. Applying oils and lotions to a stretching body can be wonderful when combined with therapeutic massage. Massage stimulates circulation along the skin surface. Depending upon what is used in the massage, the process can actually feed and nourish your skin. Taut muscles usually relax under skilled hands and the feeling of being nurtured is greatly enhanced by touch. Lymphatic fluid and blood are stimulated to flow.

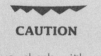

CAUTION

Always check with your doctor, nurse midwife, or other health care provider before embarking on a massage therapy program.

Plain nutritious base oils such as sweet almond or avocado can be applied at any time to keep your skin soft and oiled. During the latter stages, you can add a few drops of carefully selected pure essential oils to the base. Please check with your doctor, nurse, midwife, or aromatherapist before embarking on a massage therapy routine.

Preventing stretch marks. I wasn't aware of pure essential oils when I conceived my daughter 16 years ago. Now I often wonder how I ever coped without them. I was fortunate not to have acquired too much evidence of stretch marks. Some women are plagued with them everywhere; others have them just on the belly or hips. Genetic predisposition is the biggest factor in determining who gets stretch marks. Even without

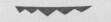

THE BENEFITS OF PRENATAL MASSAGE

Maternal prenatal massage can be traced back to ancient India, Asia, Russia, and the Middle East. The American Indians as well as settlers employed this practice. It has been found that prenatal massage even helps to calm baby while in the womb as well as the mother-to-be. Touch in the form of massage is a powerful under-utilized tool that should be used to assist life's most exciting process: the development and emergence of a new life.

Patricia B. Smith of Natal Kneads in Southfield, Michigan (see resource list) notes that pregnant women frequently report an increase in heartburn, backaches, swollen ankles, aching muscles, fatigue, and psychological stress symptoms. Physicians are often at a loss on how to deal with these because medication is general-ly contraindicated at this time. Massage is a great complimenta-ry therapy to help deal with these nagging problems that often get in the way of everyday activities.

Prenatal massage therapy can:

◆ Relieve stress by activating the relaxation response and help to stabilize hormone levels
◆ Increase circulation, which brings greater nutrition to the tissues and relieving fatigue
◆ Increase circulating red blood cells by pushing the blood vessel linings back into the blood stream, helping to lessen fatigue
◆ Increase lymphatic circulation, resulting in more energy and less edema (water weight gain)
◆ Decrease strain on the muscles of the low back, abdomen, and shoulders

Natal Kneads uses an innovative recessed cushion system allowing the pregnant woman to lie face down in comfort while receiving the full benefits of massage therapy. The massage oil combines essential oils from aromatic plants like grapefruit, laven-der, bergamot, and tangerine in a base oil to help lift your spirits and relax you. Check out your community today, you may have some great massage therapists like Pat Smith just waiting to make your Natal Kneads a reality.

essential oil knowledge, I religiously applied body oils and lotions throughout my pregnancy. The increase in circulation and the emollient action of various topical applications helped my skin stay pliable.

STRETCH MARK MASSAGE OIL

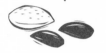

5 tablespoons base oil (one possible combination: 3 tablespoons sweet almond oil and 2 table-spoons avocado oil)
20 drops (total) of a combination of the following essential oils:
   Mandarin
   Neroli
   Tangerine

The scent of this oil blend reminds me of drives through the Florida citrus country, breathing deeply to take in the scent of the flowering orange trees on the night air. It is soothing, gentle, and delightful. Only a few drops are ever needed and, given the expense of the oils, that's all most of us can really afford to use at a time.

The citrus scents of these oils are lightly refreshing, yet mild, soothing, and calming. Both mandarin and tangerine have been safely used by clients in massage and bath oils for both moms and kids.

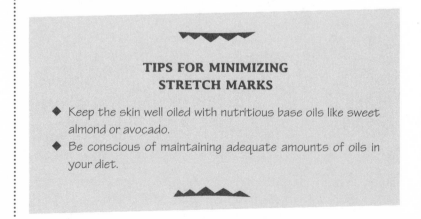

TIPS FOR MINIMIZING STRETCH MARKS

◆ Keep the skin well oiled with nutritious base oils like sweet almond or avocado.
◆ Be conscious of maintaining adequate amounts of oils in your diet.

Herbal Teas

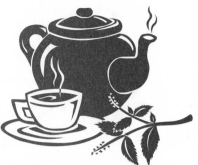

Peppermint, chamomile, and red raspberry herb teas are the best to use during pregnancy. Tea bags of varying appeal line health food shops awaiting your discovery. Many fine herb teas can be purchased by the box at the nearest health food store or through the mail.

Exercise

Check with your doctor or midwife for specific exercises that will benefit you while you're pregnant. Pelvic floor muscle exercises can aid delivery and should be incorporated into every woman's life as part of a daily routine. As women age or bear many children, muscles often become lax. Use them or lose

A NOTE ON STORE-BOUGHT PRODUCTS

It doesn't require a lot of time to take care of yourself naturally during pregnancy. If your days are full with work and other activities, don't worry that you can't make your own essential oil blends. There are many fine products available in natural food stores and even drugstores.

When buying any product, check the contents carefully to be sure they do not contain any additives or chemical preservatives to extend shelf life. Many products make claims of being "natural," "herbal," or "used for aromatherapy," but don't be fooled by these terms. There is no official standard by which they can be labeled as such. Products that claim to be useful for aromatherapy may actually contain none or very little pure essential oils.

Check out any product before you use it on yourself or your child. "Natural" holds no guarantees. Making your own blends at home or purchasing them from a reputable supplier is preferable to playing Russian roulette with all of the lotions and potions that line the store shelves.

them. Make a habit of being aware of your personal muscle strengths and weaknesses.

Be aware of how you move. As you grow throughout your pregnancy, take stock of your center of gravity. Walk as much as possible and for as long as you can comfortably. A chiropractor can help keep the spine in alignment as your body grows. This will enable your back to better carry the extra weight. You can also alleviate back pain and reduce the chance of painful problems later by learning the proper ways of moving, bending, lifting. Be aware of how you move. For instance, twisting your body as you get in and out of a car can put a real strain on the back. Becoming more conscious of your movements and learning not to swivel your body before stepping in or out of the car seat will help prevent injury.

Kegal exercises. Ask your midwife, nurse, or doctor about Kegel exercises. These internal voluntary muscular contractions that you perform yourself can help keep the muscles that help support the female organs in good shape. They can be done anytime, anywhere with no one knowing what you're up to. I also exercise this area by starting and stopping the flow of urine to help flex internal often ignored or forgotten muscles. These practices will be of service later in life when these muscles began to weaken.

Yoga. The value of yoga for pregnant women is wonderfully expressed in *Inner Beauty, Inner Light* (see reading list). In this powerful book, Frederick Leboyer leads us through the yoga practice of a young woman named Vanita, the daughter of B.K.S. Iyengar, a great yoga master. Vanita was very close to her own child's birth at the time the photographs in this book were taken.

Yoga can be a beneficial and profoundly peaceful way to tone the body and mind. As Maria Rosenstone eloquently puts it in this book, "When the intelligence of the body is awakened, as through the practice of yoga, it will guide the woman throughout the pregnancy, making her feel perhaps more in touch with her self than ever before. She is close to her own nature and ready to flow with the movement of birth when it begins."

She goes on: "The sublime energy that, when trusted to pass freely, will move the womb to open and empty itself, bringing forth the new life, will also sweep through the being of the mother, giving rise to birth and rebirth simultaneously and at each instant. The intensity of childbirth brings the supreme moment in which the usual hold on one's self can be shaken and undone. One falls into the exultation of life as it lives itself. Birth then is the occasion of vibrating with the universal rhythm, a moment to feel the perfect accord of what is below with what is above, a merging with the cosmic dance."

It's helpful to continue yoga once you're a mother as well; it can give you a few moments of peace, which may be all a mother can expect to experience in a day. Find a teacher whose approach feels right for you. Ask around, check community education classes, natural foods stores, co-ops, or holistic practitioners for listings of teachers in your area.

Tai chi. An ancient Chinese art, tai chi is a series of steps and graceful movements done in a specific order according to specific descriptions. It is quite simple to learn and provides great benefits in helping build the ability to focus the mind and body. It is a dance with the self that enables one to achieve a balance and inner harmony. Check local community education brochures for classes or private instruction in this gentle yet powerful traditional exercise.

Dreaming

Pregnant women often have very vivid, lucid dreams. Pay attention to them because they may tell a story. Keep a notepad and

---

BELLY MASK: APPRECIATING THE BEAUTY OF YOUR BODY

Lisa Forester of Better Beginnings Midwifery Services (see source list), offers pregnant women a unique way of recognizing and commemorating the beauty of their bodies during pregnancy — making belly masks. This is a plaster cast of your belly. The resulting mask is painted, and often decorated with feathers and beads. It can be hung in a nursery or home.

This unique piece of art allows a woman to see a 3-D view of her pregnant belly, usually seen from a vantage point above or in the mirror. Lisa says this mask-making process can be a moving, powerful experience, a way of creating memory of your baby within and appreciating your changing self through this process. It adds to dad's memory as well!

pencil or small recorder by your bedside so you can easily write down or record what you remember when you wake. I am so surprised when I read old records I kept of my night adventures to see how often the dreams have manifested themselves in the present.

It is not unusual for pregnant women to have frightening dreams. Our fears often come out to play in our dreams, where we are safe to experience them. Do not worry too much about a bad or scary dream; just look for helpful messages it may contain and then let it go.

Although not pregnant, I dreamt recently that I gave birth to a child with great ease and little discomfort. I was telling my daughter how easy it was and holding my baby close in complete harmony and happiness. Dream books explain birth dreams as representing a rebirth of the dreamer. I am at a time in my life where this interpretation makes perfect sense.

LABOR AND CHILDBIRTH

Birth is no longer a rather hasty, unplanned trip to the hospital, a nervous thrust-aside partner, and little regard for the mother's experience. Birth is not an illness: It is a natural progression that can be greatly enhanced by the right choice of location, surroundings, assistants and procedures. Remember, this is your birth experience not anyone else's. These memories will stay with you, your family, and your child for your entire lifetime. You can make informed birthing decisions ahead of time that will help ensure the best possible care available to you.

Today, mothers have many choices in birthing options and the attendants they want to be with them throughout the experience. Explore your choices through childbirth education classes at your local hospital, birthing center, or midwives organization (see source list). Many of these organizations have internet access so you can learn more about various options right from the comfort of your own home. Giving birth is certainly not an exact science and unexpected circumstances may well arise. However, this is a very important time for you and your mate and you are entitled to state your needs, desires, and wishes and find just the right people to support you in your decisions.

I spent one afternoon searching about birth-support organizations and individuals within a 50-mile radius of my home in Michigan. I was amazed at how much help there is available. All you have to do is ask! I sincerely hope you have as much luck as I did in finding the assistance you and your mate need.

Labor Massage

Although giving birth is one of the most special times of our lives, we need support and tender loving care whenever possible to enable our little ones to come into this world in a nurturing manner. Massage can provide soothing respite in a time racked with upheaval and stress. Pure essential oils can help relieve some of the common anxieties associated with labor and childbirth.

The role of a coach, midwife, or loved one who accompanies you through labor can be greatly enhanced by therapeutic massage. He or she can offer gentle strokes wherever you are experiencing pain, such as the small of the back. Try to visit a massage therapist or attend a class with your partner prior to your delivery date to learn some useful massage techniques.

The value of using essential oils in labor has been recognized for centuries. The simple application of an aromatic compress on the brow of a woman laboring has long been recognized as a gentle yet effective aid to relaxation and balance. Try using selected pure essential oils in a simmer pot during very relaxing times throughout your pregnancy; employ these same oils during labor to remind you to relax at a time when it is of the utmost importance.

Clary sage should be avoided during pregnancy, but labor is the time when this essential oil comes into its own. It is believed to induce and strengthen contractions and reduce stress and tension. This helps in an all-around way: Less stress means less tension, less tension means less pain, and less pain means a more relaxed, joyous birthing experience. Lisa Forester, of the Better Beginnings birthing center, reports good results from labor baths and massages using clary sage combined with lavender. She says arnica massage oil also works well for labor massage. *Note:* Clary sage is a potent essential oil that must never be used with alcohol since that may over-intensify its effects.

Labor Bath

The birthing center at Better Beginnings also uses a bath of dried herbs, including comfrey, uva ursi, sea salt, shepherd's purse, and myrrh, combined with sea salt for both baby and mom about one hour after birth. The bath is prepared by simmering the herbs to make a tea which is then strained into a tub of warm water. Mom and baby relax together in this herbal antiseptic, regenerating, cleansing, astringent bath.

You must conserve your energy for labor and birth. To avoid expending too much of your energy in anxiety and fear, you may want to try a soothing aromatic bath as you approach delivery time, if your midwife or doctor agree. I vividly recall my pre-birth soak into the wee hours. I soaked in the tub up until two hours before my daughter's birth. I feel this helped to relax me and make my bottom a bit more pliable for the stretching of labor and birth. I soaked up until the last minute and loved it. Lilacs and lily-of-the-valley scented the air and made

LABOR MASSAGE OIL

1 tablespoon of base oil
1 drop of jasmine absolute

To apply, gently massage oil into the small of the back.

The sweet fragrance of precious jasmine absolute has a calming and relaxing effect that helps to instill confidence during labor. Very little is needed (and is all you will want to use given the cost!). This oil can make a big difference in a labor room no matter if it is your own bedroom or a hospital birthing or labor room. The birth attendants will also be in for a treat when they come into contact with heavenly Jasmine Absolute: it will help revive their courage and confidence when they need it to relay to you.

me feel new and refreshed to this day. Lavender, neroli, jasmine absolute, or clary sage essential oils are all suitable for a labor bath. I meditated and welcomed my child's spirit into the world. I practiced my breathing. I washed and braided my hair and oiled my stretched body. A cup or two of hot, labor-prompting herbs, and I was ready for the most important event of my life. I had a focal point of a baby on a wooden and leather necklace that I used to concentrate on during labor. It said, "The Creator's Creation." It still hangs in my room.

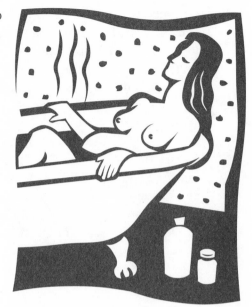

I left my house at 4:00 A.M. and Christina was born at 6:11 A.M. I purposely wanted to avoid spending any more time in the hospital than I needed to, since I don't like the smell or the scrutiny under which one is placed there. I know that for some mothers the care provided by a medical staff is essential, and hopefully you will have assistants that are willing to cooperate with your personal wishes. Make your needs known as soon as possible. You have specific rights and choices. Ask questions and be in control of your birthing experience. If you must hurry along to the hospital, pre-pack your labor massage oil, rescue remedy (dad may need some too!), and your favorite focal point.

Labor Bath Salts

If you are healthy, and your labor coach, doctor, or midwife agrees, by all means have a nice warm soak before the rigors of birth. However, *never* soak in a tub if your water has broken. For a heavenly soak, add the entire 1-pint to a tubful of warm water. If a bath tub is unavailable, try a footbath with ½ pint of bath salts in a basin of warm water. Encourage your birthing assistants to take a soak with one of these salt combinations after they assist you in your miracle!

The essential oil combinations used in these salt blends can also be used to make aromatic compresses for use during labor. Simply add the pure essential oils to a basin of warm water, mix well, and dip a small cotton cloth in. Apply to the lower back, abdomen, or head. Use caution, however, because sometimes the undiluted essential oils cling to the cloth, so always fold the dipped side away from direct skin contact and make sure pure essential oils are well dispersed in the water. Watch the rainbows and oil slicks form, and dance upon the water and releasing their precious essence all the while. Some disperse quite quickly, others linger or fall to the bottom. The oils could also be added to a tablespoon of base oil and used to lightly massage wherever the expectant mother needs it.

BATH SALTS COMBINATION #1

1 pint sea salt
1 drop clary sage essential oil
1 drop jasmine absolute
1 drop lavender essential oil

BATH SALTS COMBINATION #2

1 pint sea salt
1 drop clary sage essential oil
1 drop rose otto essential oil
1 drop neroli (orange blossom) essential oil

BATH SALTS COMBINATION #3

1 pint sea salt
1 drop rose otto essential oil
1 drop sandalwood essential oil
1 drop ylang-ylang essential oil

BATH SALTS COMBINATION #4

1 pint sea salt
1 drop rose absolute or otto
1 drop clary sage essential oil
1 drop sandalwood essential oil

Combine the salt and essential oils in a bowl and blend well so oils are well diluted and any lumps are well crushed. Store in a 1-pint canning jar.

BREASTFEEDING

Few issues bring up such emotional outcries as that of how a woman decides to feed her offspring. The feeding of infants has undergone many changes throughout history — from the use of wet nurses to high-tech breast pumps. Bottle feeding enjoyed a tenacious hold in our society up until the 1980s and the medical community often discouraged nursing. Valerie Fildes in her book *Breasts, Bottles, and Babies,* details this evolution through history, and Rima D. Apple takes us from 1890 to 1950 in her book *Mothers and Medicine* (see reading list).

Many think breastfeeding should just come naturally, that women have an innate knowledge when it comes to infant feeding. This may be true in theory but, rewarding as the experience is, it isn't always so easy as just putting a child to the breast. Breastfeeding can be challenging in physical, emotional, and social ways. You can run into a variety of problems, from a painful clogged milk duct to a baby who can't seem to get the hang of latching on. There are *no* dumb questions, except for the ones not asked and addressed.

Formula feeding has its place, and you don't need to feel guilty if you must forgo breastfeeding. But please inquire about help. I always felt a profound comfort being my child's main source of food. The milk she had was always at the perfect temperature, readily available, and came in decorative containers. Sure, sometimes I wondered if she would nurse until she was 10 or if my breasts would end up in my lap by the time she was finished nursing, but I am happy to report that neither has happened. I saved valuable time and energy by not having to wash bottles or mix formula. I did, however, have to watch my diet, and was picky about products I ingested or put upon my body. In a world of open sexuality I feel we have lost sight of the purpose breasts have. I hope you take the time to research breastfeeding.

A Personal Experience

My daughter was born at dawn, 6:11 A.M., on Good Friday April 4, 1980. I always knew I wanted to breastfeed. The main obstacle I experienced was lack of information and support.

When I was nursing my daughter, I was basically on my own. I asked to be left alone with her in my hospital room, and insisted she be left with me and not returned to the nursery, where I feared she would be given supplemental feedings of glucose water, which I thought would surely interfere with her desire to nurse when she was brought to me. I was treated like a problem radical in the hospital, and knowing what I know now I would have certainly opted for a home or birthing-center birth if possible.

I had to fight to keep her with me right after she was born. The nurses repeatedly told me I needed to rest; I insisted I needed to bond with and nurse my child. I went home as soon as possible; in fact, I packed her up and brought her home on Easter Sunday. The nurses were right, I did need my rest, but I needed to rest with my daughter at my breast.

Oh, how I recall the swollen breasts that I would sometimes pump out in a hot shower just to obtain relief. I remember the reflex that triggers the letdown of milk that left me soaked with my own milk in odd places at odd times when I would hear a baby cry or think of my little one at home with Dad or a close friend. Sex was a damp adventure, indeed, as orgasm often stimulated the letdown reflex and generated enough milk to feed us all.

I was truly amazed at the capacity of my breasts to measure and dole out just enough milk, and how unbalanced I would feel when the baby fell asleep after nursing on only one side. There were times when I felt trapped and thought she would nurse until she went to school. There were also moments at sunrise or in the night when I would hold my dear little one to my breast and know a profound peace. Our nursing periods were the most wonderful. The strong and loving bond we forged lasts to this day, and I am grateful that I had the opportunity to experience the art of breastfeeding. When my daughter would look at me and say, "Nur-nur, Momma, nur-nur," my heart would melt and I felt I had permission to sit or lie down for a short respite from the world and enjoy being a woman and a mother. The belief that I was giving her the best possible start in life was deeply satisfying, and an experience whose memory can tickle my heart to this day.

Find a Support Group

When I was breastfeeding, I was lucky enough to find support through the La Leche League (see resources), and from a group of moms like me who wanted to give their children nature's best whenever possible. Many women find much-needed support from groups that meet in local hospitals, doctors' offices, midwives' associations, community houses, or through their health care plans. Reach out: As I mentioned before there are no rewards for being brave or uninformed. You may meet many fine people who will remain in the lives of you and your children for many years.

The invaluable experience of those who have gone before us is a treasure. I don't know if I could have always held my own when outsiders gave me those stares that said, "My God, is she really nursing a baby under that blanket?" Or the well-meaning comment, "My dear, don't you think she's getting too old to still be nursing?" I heard remarkable stories of women who nursed adopted babies, handicapped babies, and even after intense personal medical challenges. I quickly realized I was not alone, and that help was often only a few blocks away.

I still have contact with the women and young folks who were part of our life during pregnancy and birth. My neighbor and former La Leche League colleague Sue Greba, R.N., and I have maintained a relationship since our children were babies. When I see her children, and the young adult children of other La Leche League sisters, I can't help but have a little smile in my heart for them. Today, the mothers provide encouragement to each other as we watch our "babies" move away from us and into young lives of their own. These are invaluable ties that make a community a better place to live, work, and grow. Sue took her interest in breastfeeding a huge step further by becoming one of the first certified lactation consultants in this area.

Tips for Better Breastfeeding

Here are some basic tips for a better breastfeeding experience from Sue Greba, R.N., IBCLC (International Board Certified Lactation Consultant). She works for a Michigan hospital, teaches classes, and attends health fairs in her quest to educate women about breastfeeding.

1. Educate yourself.

Attend prenatal breast-feeding classes and La Leche League meetings (call 1-800-LA LECHE for a free catalog) before and after delivery. There isn't usually much time to talk with a trained lactation consultant in the hospital or if you opt for a home birth, so following up yourself is very important to success. If you go home from the hospital in less than 48 hours, your baby needs to be seen by a doctor two to three days after discharge and again after ten days to two weeks for a physical assessment and weight check. It is your responsibility to schedule these office visits and let your doctor or certified lactation consultant know then if you feel breastfeeding is not going well.

2. Nurse as soon as possible after delivery.

The baby is most alert the first hour after delivery, after that he or she will want to go into much-needed rest. The sooner the baby nurses, the sooner your milk will come in. Colostrum that is present in the first nursing session has a laxative effect which will help the baby stool and be effective at keeping jaundice at bay. The sooner you nurse, the sooner your confidence is built that you can feed this child on your own. This also stimulates the uterine contractions and keeps bleeding to a minimum.

3. Make sure your baby is positioned and latched on to the breast correctly.

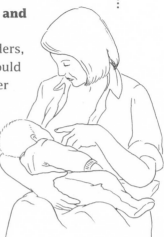

The baby should be aligned so that the shoulders, hips, and ears line up straight. The baby should be tummy to tummy with the mother. His or her mouth should be wide open and the nose should touch the breast. The lips should be flanged out and you should be able to see movement around the baby's ears or the top of the jawline. If nursing is painful, the baby is probably not positioned correctly. Intense pain is not normal. Have a trained professional help you as soon as possible if you are experiencing pain. Incorrect nursing procedures can cause sore nipples that can take days to heal.

Ask questions: Don't assume that just because you're a woman, you should automatically know how to nurse. Childbirth is natural, yet we need assistance and often the voice of experience to establish correct practices and avoid unnecessary pain. Be patient with yourself and your baby. Breastfeeding is a learned technique that takes several weeks to properly establish.

4. Feed the baby often.

If your child has slept more than three or four hours, wake him or her to feed. Look for any cues the baby is ready to eat such as opening the mouth or bringing the hands to the mouth. Be aware of signs that your baby is more alert or wants to nurse. Most babies cluster feed, wanting to eat a lot for a period of time and then sleeping. Babies should demand to eat at least eight to twelve times a day, but these feedings may not be at regular intervals or at the same time everyday.

After a few weeks your baby will develop his or her own style and schedule. Remember, happy babies make happy parents! It's better for you to adjust to the baby's schedule than to try to train such a young child to fit your schedule.

5. Try to avoid using bottles unless medically indicated.
Babies suck differently on a bottle than on a breast and may be confused by the mixture. If your baby needs to have a supplement, try using an eyedropper, syringe, or small cup. Whenever possible, use breast milk. Water is not necessary for a newborn who is learning to nurse. It doesn't lessen jaundice; in fact, it can actually increase the possibility. If you want to supplement feedings, wait a few weeks until lactation is firmly established so you can better maintain your nursing relationship. Bottles indicate an actual start of weaning of the baby. Breast milk is a complete food for most babies for the first six months without any supplementation.

6. How do you know if baby is getting enough to eat?
Milk should be flowing from your breasts by day four after delivery. Your breasts should be fuller or heavier and show leakage. You should be able to hear your baby swallow and gulp. The baby should have at least six to eight wet diapers a day that are soaked, odorless, and clear. Baby should also start having breast-fed stools which are loose, yellow, and explosive (oh, fun!). Breast-fed babies don't burp too well, so passing gas

HERBS THAT AID IN MILK PRODUCTION

The following herbs are known to increase milk flow in a nursing mom: fennel, borage (which grows wild in abundance every year in my gardens), basil (make pesto!), marshmallow fenugreek (which can be sprouted for salads), and hops (I drank an occasional organically brewed beer whenever I could find one when I was nursing; *occasional* and *one* are key here).

To decrease milk production try making a tea with garden sage, adding ½ teaspoon garden sage to 1 cup boiling water, covering, and steeping for 5 minutes. You may also add ½ teaspoon red raspberry leaf, peppermint, lemon balm, or chamomile.

is perfectly normal. Some breast-fed babies have a bowel movement at each feeding, some have only one once a day; it should always be loose, never formed.

If your baby is at birthweight or more by two weeks old this indicates successful breastfeeding (along with the indicators mentioned above).

Breast Care

Air and sunlight exposure is good for your breasts. It builds up a keratin layer over the nipple that looks like dry skin or is very shiny. This helps protect the nipples from becoming sore. Breast milk is good for nipples. Rub it on after feedings and let your nipples air dry.

Wearing a supportive bra is very important to overall breast health. Avoid excessive soaps and lotions on the breasts since they can remove the protective keratin layer. If your nipples are cracked or bleeding, you should seek immediate attention from a certified lactation consultant or midwife.

Engorgement is a temporary condition that exists when milk first comes in. Heat and massage will help soften the breasts; feeding the baby often, at least every two hours, will also help relieve this condition. A plugged duct can aggravate a staph infection that may lead to mastitis if left untreated. Mastitis could be indicated by flu-like symptoms including high temperature, warm reddened area on the breast, and pain. Heat, rest, and emptying the breast (by continual nursing) help relieve this condition. You should seek medical attention as well since antibiotics may be necessary.

CARING FOR YOURSELF DURING THE POSTPARTUM OR POSTNATAL PERIOD

As I recall, immediately following my daughter's birth the world seemed a more beautiful place. The sun shone brighter, the air smelled sweeter, and the whole Earth sang the song of spring. I was full of energy after her birth. I didn't even sleep for the first 24 hours after she was born. I came home, cleaned house, cooked food, and then fell into a deep sleep, my daughter at my side.

Minimizing Postpartum Depression

While I didn't experience much postpartum depression, I was stressed and a little bewildered by the new body I was left with, along with the responsibility of feeding an infant in addition to running a home. My stepson, who was eight years old, was a great help. I suggest the following actions for getting through the adjustments of the postpartum period.

Arrange for help. Do this before you give birth, if possible. New mothers are sent home from the hospital so soon now — and many opt to forgo a hospital stay entirely — that there's little time for them to catch their breath before launching into their new childcare responsibilities. You're going to need and appreciate help with child care, running errands, cooking, and cleaning.

Allow yourself the freedom to ask for help. There is no merit badge awarded for toughing it out yourself. For a new mom in distress, a listening ear or the offer of a heartfelt hug can make all the difference. Once you're through this period, offer to do the same for another new mom.

I have found that neighbors can be a benefit at those odd times when you just need to go out for a few moments to the pharmacy or grocery and packing up the baby seems a lot of work if you are weary. Especially if there are other young children at home, this little adventure could take hours. I always

---

Product Tip
RELAXATION TAPES

Look for tools that will help guide you into relaxation. Tape recordings such as "Relax and Enjoy Your Baby: A Complete Program of Relaxation for New and Expectant Parents" can help ease your stress. Created by The Relaxation Company (see resource list), this tape by childbirth educator Sylvia Klein Olkin offers a series of short guided relaxation exercises, some geared specifically to moms and others specifically to dads. The background music used on these tapes has been found to have a soothing effect on infants in utero.

hated taking a sick child into a pharmacy if prescriptions were absolutely necessary.

Rest. Lie down every chance you get. When the baby is sleeping, try to take a nap yourself. The dishes will wait; your energy level will only be less if you work the entire time the baby rests. Being divorced when my daughter was young made this advice hard for me to follow. I always tried "to get something done" while she slept and found myself worn out when she was just getting going again.

Even when you don't have the chance to actually lie down, try to relax. The homeopathic Bach Rescue Remedy can be helpful when you're feeling overwhelmed or out of control. If you've got a willing partner or friend, accept a relaxing neck and shoulder massage with a few drops of Roman chamomile and/or lavender essential oils combined with a base oil.

Eat well. Skimping on your diet means skimping on your ability to keep up with the demands of parenting. Eating well provides adequate nourishment to enable us to carry on. Don't be concerned about losing weight (right!) if you can help it — this is not the time to worry about losing, but a time to rebuild.

Especially if you are nursing your child, you'll need all the energy you can muster just to keep up with that demand on your body. When you make something particularly yummy, can or freeze some of the dish for the days when you just don't have the time to cook. If friends want to know how they can help, ask them to prepare a meal in their home and deliver it to yours. Tell them how grateful you are for this luxury, and reciprocate when you can.

Drink plenty of fluids. Lots of pure water is a must, every day. Carry it in the diaper bag as part of your essentials. Dilute pure juices with fresh water. Herb teas, especially if they are right out of the garden, are invaluable for a new mother's health.

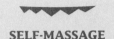

SELF-MASSAGE

To calm yourself through difficult times, self-massage can be very beneficial. Just one drop of lavender or Roman chamomile essential oil diluted in one tablespoon of sweet almond oil makes a nice massage mixture that you can carry in a small bottle tucked into the pocket of a diaper bag or purse. When you're feeling stressed, take a few minutes to relax and massage this oil into your skin. Enjoy the experience as the essence is slowly diffused from the skin. If you're nursing, avoid the nipple area or cleanse well after massage.

To make your own herb tea, simply add 1 cup of hot water to ½ to 1 teaspoon of fresh herbs. Chamomile, red raspberry leaf, and fennel are all good herb teas for nursing mothers. Garden sage is useful if you are trying to dry up your milk (see box on page 64).

▼▼▼▼▼

Product tip
HERBAL TEAS

You'll find teas in many supermarkets and at health food stores that contain herbs that aid in producing milk or calming mother. These are packaged in convenient bags that are easy to carry along if you are eating away from home. The company Traditional Medicinals offers teas with names such as Mother's Milk, Pregnancy Tea, Women's Liberty, PMS Tea, Female Toner, and Raspberry Leaf in take-along tea bags.

▲▲▲▲

Get enough exercise. One of the main concerns for new mothers is how to fit in time for exercise. If you think about it, you may be surprised by how many opportunities we have to work out in the process of daily living, while performing tasks from laundry to gardening.

Squatting is a great form of exercise. I keep the basket of laundry on the ground, with the wooden clothespins in it as well. I squat to pick up the clothes, squat for a clothespin, and squat to put a dry, folded piece back in the basket. When doing laundry indoors, I squat down to the dryer door instead of bending down.

While gardening a few days ago, I actually counted how many squats I did in a four-hour period — approximately 500! I squatted when I planted seedlings, loaded mulch into a wheelbarrow, placed the mulch around the plants and then rocks around the mulch. I probably never would have done these deep knee bends just as an exercise. My muscles are gently stretched and strengthened every time I squat and rise up again. They feel much stronger than they did a month ago, before gardening season.

I also keep things on shelves high enough that I gain a gentle stretch in my upper body while reaching for items I use daily.

Walking is the easiest and most stress-reducing exercise I know. I am fortunate to live by a lake that I can walk around. Surrounded by woods, I have a haven to travel through while gaining strength and sorting out mental tasks. In summer I often walk at night (exercise personal caution here; be aware of your surroundings). In parking lots I leave my car in the most distant spaces; that way, I get exercise walking to stores. Think about other methods of incorporating gentle exercise into your daily routine.

Consider how you physically handle your child's weight while carrying him or her. Try to develop good habits in how you lift and carry a child, especially as he grows heavier. The way you lift, bend, squat, twist, and even get in and out of your car has an impact on your muscle and skeletal systems. Notice how you move. Make a mental note to respect any little aches or twinges in muscle or bone. These are signals not to be ignored. Try to begin moving a little slower and more deliberately. If you can, take a class in yoga, tai chi, or other movement and body awareness exercise to become more conscious of how you move and how to increase your own comfort as you do so.

Natural Menstrual Care

If you're like most women, you probably don't think too much about the products you use to absorb menstrual flow or discharge after birth. We go to the store, buy our favorite brand, and enjoy the convenience of disposable menstrual aids. Tampons and pads are available with wings, in various shapes, absorbencies, and deodorized. They appear white, sanitary, and safe. Well, think again! You might want to consider what women did for centuries when menstrual protection wasn't as easy as a trip to the local drugstore. I was told once by an older woman that when she was younger she found men's fresh, white cotton socks were her pad of choice. Some of you are squirming in your seat, saying, "Yuck, I wouldn't want to deal with stained pads or reusable ones." I remember laughing at the term "recycled toilet paper." Well, perhaps you'd rather deal with dioxin.

Dioxin is a chemical compound present in tampons, menstrual pads, and disposable diapers. An article in *Mothering Magazine,* Summer 1993 entitled "Dioxin in Single-Use Diapers and Tampons," gives an alarming report on this and other chemicals found in these products. There is increasing evidence that dioxin is much more dangerous than was previously believed.

In 1980, the Centers for Disease Control reported 812 menstrual cases of toxic shock syndrome, including 42 deaths. Toxic shock is attributed to bacteria not chemicals, but I can't help but wonder if the two are interrelated.

The ads for mass-marketed feminine products portray soft, flowery, stress-free care. Nothing could be farther from the truth. I often warn about the use of synthetic fragrances and perfumes, yet many women use deodorant tampons every month. In *Whitewash,* authors Liz Armstrong and Adrienne Scott give a thorough account of the dioxin concerns we must address (see reading list).

In an article in *Buzzworm,* a bimonthly environmental journal, entitled "With Strings Attached," Marina Lindsey cites a 1980 finding published in *Obstetrics & Gynecology* that chemical fragrances in deodorant tampons can cause internal irritation and disrupt a woman's microbial balance. There are no federal regulations known to me that control the levels of toxic chemicals used to produce sanitary protection products or single-use diapers. Furthermore, neither of these products is even sterile.

There are natural alternatives available that are soft, comfortable, washable, reusable products. I have used cotton pads for many years. The comfort is unbeatable. I can actually feel a great difference when I succumb to using a commercial pad. I wholeheartedly suggest you look into this natural alternative. Put the money you would spend on menstrual products into a

CALMING PRE-MENSTRUAL CRAMPS

Clary Sage, often used to tone and stimulate the uterus, can help ease the tension of rough pre-menstrual days.

Simmer pot: Add 2 drops clary sage essential oil to a simmer pot of water placed by your bedside while you rest.

Mild massage oil: Add 1 drop of clary sage essential oil to 1 tablespoon base oil such as sweet almond and rub on the belly. You can also add 1 drop of chamomile and/or lavender if you like.

fund and do something wonderful for yourself with it, or donate to an environmentally friendly association. For centuries, women have gotten along without toxic products to aid them in a completely natural process. Please don't give in to the shame-based advertising for these potentially dangerous products. Do some research, then tell your friends and your daughters.

PAMPERING YOURSELF

One of the most important ways you can care for yourself and help ensure you'll be the best parent you can be is to make time for your own mental and physical health. Of course, you don't have much time. But nature's pantry provides an abundance of ingredients to enhance your life: body, mind, and spirit. Become aware that you can make choices to enhance your well-being personally which will of course be all the better for your baby and whole family.

HERBS AND THEIR EFFECTS

Stimulating and Refreshing

Basil
Lemongrass
Nettle
Peppermint
Rose geranium
Rosemary
Spearmint

Refreshing

Chamomile
Clary sage
Lavender
Lemon balm
Linden or lime blossoms
Rose
Sage

Other Uses

Calendula (skincare)
Comfrey (skincare)
Horsetail (strengtens nails and hair)
Lady's mantle (skincare)
Oatmeal (soothing and regenerating for skin)
Patchouli (skincare)
Red clover (blood cleanser; facial steams; hair rinses; herb baths)
Thyme (antiseptic)
Yarrow (astringent tea applied locally for hemorrhoids)

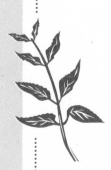

You can turn just a few minutes a day into a luxurious experience that will have beneficial results. With a few herbs, essential oils, base oils, lotions, sea salt, or favorite unscented body cream, you can easily create an aromatic paradise in your own home.

Some Simple Herbal Beauty Recipes

Herb concoctions have been used to enhance women's beauty routines for centuries. These were referred to as "simples." Using herbs and essential oils in everyday life need not be difficult or inconvenient. A few basic herbs either grown in the garden or purchased by the ounce from a reputable supplier can turn your bathroom into an aromatic spa. The only equipment you'll need is a nonaluminum pan (to avoid any chemical reactions) and a fine-mesh tea strainer.

I've included a few easy recipes here. There are some great books you can use to explore the world of herbal beauty listed in the reading list.

EASY FACIAL OR BODY SCRUB

⅓ cup whole oats
Water

Place the oatmeal into a coffee grinder and grind it up very fine. For a facial, combine a tablespoon of this ground oatmeal with enough water to make a paste. Apply to face and *gently* scrub the skin. Rinse well with warm water. Use more oatmeal for a full body scrub.

If desired, you can add 1 teaspoon of herbs to the grinder along with the oatmeal to meet your individual skin-care needs. For dry skin, add rose or calendula. For oily skin, add lemongrass or rosemary. For normal skin, add lavender, peppermint, or comfrey. For sensitive skin, add chamomile.

This excellent facial scrub is quick and economical to make.

SALT GLOW

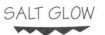

2 cups (500 ml) sea salt
1 ounce base oil
6–8 drops essential oil or
    absolute

Combine all ingredients in a bowl and mix well with your hands. Make sure to crush the little drops of oil that clump in the salt.

Stand nude in a dry bathtub and gently massage the body, starting with the feet. Work your way up, massaging in a circular, clockwise motion. As the oiled salts fall to the base of the tub, pick them up and reuse them until the entire body (except for face and neck) has been massaged. Then fill the tub with warm water and soak your cares away. The skin becomes soft, stimulated, and sweetly scented.

This recipe, from *The Essential Oils Book,* is useful for exfoliating dead skin cells on the body, although it is too harsh for the delicate skin of the face and neck. The skin literally glows after applying and bathing in this blend.

EASY FACIAL MASK

½ teaspoon kaolin clay
Water

Combine kaolin clay with enough water to make a paste. Apply mixture to the face and feel its tightening and stimulating properties.

For a relaxing mask, add 1 drop of lavender or chamomile pure essential oil to the clay and mix well before adding the water.

Kaolin clay is available in most health food stores. There are various types of clays, each with different properties. Once, when Christina was small and napping, I applied a clay mask. When she awoke and called to me, I went to her having forgotten my clay mask. She took one look at me and let out a howl. I do not think she knew it was her loving mommy under that green mask!

Herbal Baths

The promise of a soothing herbal bath got me through more than one rough day of mothering. Put a handful or two of your favorite herbs in a cloth bag, knee-high nylon, or a clean, odd sock, knot it up, and toss it in the tub for a lovely soak in a big herb tea. You can also make a bag from a cotton washcloth, fill it with a handful of herbs, and tie it with a rubber band and ribbon. Use the bag to scrub your skin and enjoy all of nature's soothing herbal properties.

Another way to prepare bath herbs is to combine 4 tablespoons of herbs with 2 to 3 quarts of water in a nonaluminum pan, cover, and simmer over low heat for 5 to 10 minutes. Pour the mixture through a strainer directly into your bathtub. Be sure to put the spent herbs on your plants or compost pile to further their usefulness.

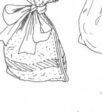

Homemade bath bag options.

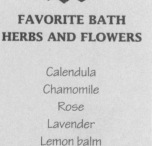

FAVORITE BATH HERBS AND FLOWERS

Calendula
Chamomile
Rose
Lavender
Lemon balm
Lemon verbena
Peppermint
Rosemary
Sage
Spearmint

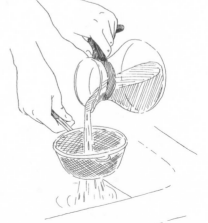

Pouring steeped herbal "tea" directly into the bath.

Hair Rinses

An herbal hair rinse can be either left in your hair or rinsed out before drying. You can also add a teaspoon or even less of your favorite hair conditioner to the base recipe for extra conditioning, and then rinse well in cool water before allowing to dry. Or you can shampoo and condition your hair as usual and then use this herbal rinse as a final rinse. Enjoy whatever works best for you. Experiment!

Nettle is an excellent addition to any hair rinse or bath recipe; however, if you harvest fresh nettles, wear your gloves — remember how they got the name of stinging nettle! What is so stinging in fresh form is mildly stimulating in dried form, or after it has been made into a "simple."

Red clover is another herb I like to add to bath and hair-rinse herb blends as well.

ESSENTIAL OIL BATH BLENDS FOR NEW MOTHERS

To make these easy baths, simply add the oils directly to a tubful of warm water and mix well before getting in. Then lie back, breathe deeply, and enjoy!

Relaxing Bath
2 drops lavender
2 drops Roman chamomile
2 drops ylang-ylang

Antidepressant Bath
2 drops bergamot
2 drops rose
2 drops grapefruit

Wake-Up Bath
2 drops rosemary
2 drops lemon
2 drops peppermint

SIMPLE HERBAL HAIR RINSE

For dark hair: 2 to 4 tablespoons of dried rosemary and dried sage (double amount if using fresh herbs)

For light hair: 2 to 4 tablespoons of chamomile and calendula petals (fresh or dried)

Add herbs to 2 cups of water in a nonaluminum pan. Cover and simmer for 5 minutes; turn off heat and let stand, covered for 5 to 10 minutes. Cool the mixture, strain, then it's ready to rinse through the hair.

Variation: Add 1 teaspoon of cider vinegar to help untangle and clarify the hair. Vinegar rinses should not be used more than once a week, however, because they can dry the hair too much.

Another vinegar hair-rinse base can be made by combining the herbs with just enough vinegar to cover in a nonmetallic container. Let sit for 2 weeks. To use, add 2 tablespoons of this base to 2 cups of warm water.

Skin Care

There are a number of good books of recipes for making your own skincare products, including *The Herbal Body Book* by Stephanie Tourles, *The Natural Soap Book* by Susan Miller Cavitch, and *Natural Beauty Illustrated* by Liz Earle (see reading list). For balm recipes that are good for both mom and baby, see pages 99 to 101.

WORKING WITH FRESH HERBS

It takes a while to get used to working with fresh herbs. In earlier times, household health depended greatly upon knowledge of herbs and spices. They have a fascinating history. You may feel overwhelmed by the amount of information available on each herb. Begin by learning about a few at a time. Growing the herbs is another excellent way to get to know them (see chapter 4). With experience, you'll get to know and enjoy the refreshing spirit of the herbs, and find that the scents linger in your memory for a lifetime.

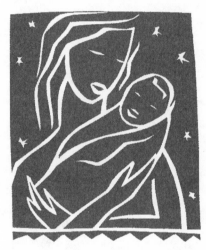

Aromababy:
Healthy Scents
for Cleaning &
Caring for Baby

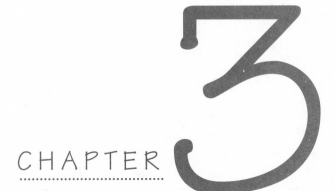

CHAPTER

When we think of caring for babies, the most immediate association for many people is the scent — baby powder, fresh baby clothes, or warm baby hair. We love the scent of popular baby products because it reminds us of the love we have for our children, or the children we are caring for.

I'm sure you've heard many people say, "I just love the scent of a baby." What do babies smell like? They smell like all that we do to nurture them, or the lack thereof. They smell like the fresh little folks that they are before all of the buildup of an often toxic lifestyle and hormone fluctuations accumulates in their bodies.

THE IMPORTANCE OF SCENT

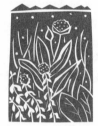 The scents with which you surround yourself and your baby will return to visit throughout your child's lifetime. Babies and children thrive on their sense of smell. They want to smell and taste everything they get their hands on. I believe it would be difficult to overemphasize the value of olfactory stimulation. Scents are our link to the world around us. The manufacturers of children's toys know this — they have known that kids are scent sensitive for longer than most parents have. "Scratch and sniff" is alive and well, and delighting kids daily. Too bad these are usually synthetic scents.

Everyone and every home has its own odor print. If you lead a naturally aromatic life, there is little or no need for perfumes or air fresheners, which are usually intended to disguise or cover up disagreeable odors. Pure essential oils and herbs actually eliminate or prevent odors; their antiseptic properties discourage bacterial growth which causes odor and their aromatic properties offer alternative, natural scents.

When you incorporate herbs and pure essential oils into your lifestyle, you develop an individually scented aura that is unique to your habits and preferences. I haven't heard of any mass-produced perfume doing that. Nature weaves an aromatic web about us that is like a guardian angel.

Comforting Scents

Our personal scent comforts our children. My daughter, Christina, taught me this lesson long ago when she was almost three years old. I was preparing to go out of town for work. I had rarely left her and she didn't like the idea of my going. I asked her what would make it easier for her to handle my absence, and explained that I had to work so that I could be home with her on most of the other days. She thought for a moment and replied that while I was gone she would like to sleep in the flannel nightdress I had worn the night before. I was happy to let her do that and proceeded to throw it into the wash basket to have all fresh and clean for her. She took it out of the basket and protested that if I washed it, then my scent would be gone from it, and that is why she wanted to sleep in it. She said it smelled like being close to me. It was then that it struck me: After nursing or being so close as a baby, a mother's scent could indeed be a comfort to a young child.

Developing an Odor Print for Your Home

In polite society it's rare to suggest that we can actually detect the scent of another. When we do, it is often a negative association. In fact, we process many scent clues from our environment in a few short seconds. How do you usually know your child needs a diaper change? Scent certainly plays a large part in the hygiene we afford ourselves, our homes, and our children. Become aware of the "odor print" in your home, and the scents you are introducing into your child's life. Wouldn't it be nicer to smell lavender or tea tree in a diaper pail instead of all the harsh chemicals that are usually used to soak diapers? You can develop your own sentimental scents for your children every day, right in your home. The next time you peel an orange, lemon, grapefruit, or lime, squeeze the peel and let a child see and smell the pure essential oils that flow out of the ruptured cells in the peel. You can even make your own kitchen spice potpourri to keep the fragrance circulating throughout your kitchen for months.

MAKE YOUR OWN
KITCHEN SPICE POTPOURRI

Approximately 2 cups of dried citrus peels such as
   orange, lemon, grapefruit, or lime*
Approximately 1 cup of any combination of the following
   herbs:
   Dried spearmint or peppermint
   Dried calendula petals
   Dried lemon verbena
   Dried geranium
   Dried lemon balm
   Dried thyme
1 cup fuzzy lamb's ears (optional)
Whole pieces of cinnamon, allspice, and cloves
1 teaspoon mixed powdered spices, including cinnamon,
   clove, allspice; or pumpkin pie spice mix
10 drops of your favorite citrus essential oils (sweet
   orange, lemon, lime, bergamot, or grapefruit) for each
   cup of dried materials

Combine the dried peel with the herbs, breaking the peel up
just prior to mixing to release the oils trapped deep inside.
Put the mixture in a jar large enough so that you can gently
turn the mixture; place out of direct light or heat, and let it
stand for 2 weeks, turning it daily. In no time you have a
lovely kitchen spice potpourri. I call mine Orange A-Peel™! For
great gifts, fill up those baby-food jars that are cluttering
the cabinets, tie a ribbon around the lids, and let a child draw
some labels.

*To dry the citrus peels, cut them into thin slices so they will not mold. Hang
them in an old onion bag in a warm, dry corner or lay them on a cookie sheet
placed in the oven with just the pilot light on and the door just ajar.

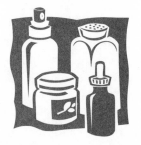

SOOTHING SKINCARE

You don't need to do much to alter the natural scent of a baby, but scents can be used to help soothe and heal in particular situations and to help create a pleasing, aromatic home environment.

Aromatic Waters

Any pure essential oil is too strong to use directly on or near a baby, but hydrosols, or floral waters, are a good alternative. Hydrosols are literally the waters used in the distillation process when pure essential oils are removed from the plant base such as lavender, chamomile, orange blossom (neroli), or rose. They contain many of the properties and characteristics of the plants (and the pure essential oils from the plants), but in a much milder form that is gentle enough to use on children.

Wiping a baby's bottom with aromatic flora waters is much nicer and kinder to your baby's skin than using synthetic baby wipes. A cotton pad moistened with aromatic water is perfect for wiping any area of your baby's skin to calm, soothe, cool, refresh, and cleanse. To calm a fussy baby, try combining rosewater with a few drops of Bach Rescue Remedy on a cotton pad and wiping the child's body. Lavender or chamomile waters are also very calming. Lavender is particularly reviving and soothing during travel. And, it works equally well for cleaning up or refreshing a frazzled parent!

I suggest carrying a fresh bottle of floral water and some small white cotton cloths, along with a plastic bag for the used ones, right along in your diaper bag. Most herbal or essential oil waters contain no preservatives, so you should only carry them in small amounts and use them, as soon as possible. Think of these natural cleanup waters as freshly made products that are perishable. Some should even be kept refrigerated to ensure freshness. Tincture of benzoin has traditionally been used as a preservative for natural products, but this is not added to floral waters because it contains a small amount of alcohol.

Making your own. Aromatic waters may be made by adding 1 to 2 drops of pure essential oil to 4 ounces (118 ml) of spring water. I like to put the mixture in a 4-ounce (118-ml) spray bottle. This mixture must be used daily or refrigerated since it does not have any preservatives in it.

Use caution when selecting the pure essential oils to use. I suggest using only lavender, chamomile, or rose otto (although this latter should be avoided during early pregnancy). Children have very delicate skin and too high a concentration could cause irritation. Start with a 1 percent dilution. While some aromatherapy experts use up to a 5 percent dilution, the knowledge required to make this judgement comes with personal experience and training. Remember, with pure essential oils less is best!

Julia Lawless's book *Lavender Oil: The New Guide to Nature's Most Versatile Remedy* is a must for the aromatherapy library (see reading list). In this little gem, she suggests that lavender is especially suited to the treatment of children because of its low toxicity level. In her companion book on rose oil, Lawless notes that restlessness, hyperactivity, and

---

Product Tip
FLORAL WATERS (HYDROSOLS)

Aromaland (see resource list) is a company that offers high-quality floral waters, including bulgarian rose, chamomile, and lavender. These products contain no drying alcohol or chemicals so they can be used safely on baby's skin.

When you select a product to use on your baby, ask yourself if you would use this product on your own face. Only use the products on your children that you would use on the most delicate parts of your own skin. For instance, would you use synthetic baby wipes to clean your own face? A mild floral water is much more appealing.

When buying rosewaters, be particularly aware of synthetic versions that many shops will call the real, pure thing.

insomnia in babies, infants, and older children can be helped by the use of rose oil in the bath or for massage.

Herbal Tisanes

Herbal tisanes or teas are made directly from fresh or dried herbs. These are much less concentrated than aromatic floral waters since they contain much less essential oil. A tisane is made just like a cup of herbal tea, in fact, a "weak tea" or infusion is another name for it. It is soothing, refreshing, inexpensive, and like a fresh herbal bath. A tisane can be used to bathe, rinse the hair, or to just sponge off a little one's body.

Research several herbs and their properties to find the ones that best suit you and your child. Some of the herbs most suitable to use in a tisane for children are: lavender to soothe the skin and calm the baby, chamomile to relax and also soothe the skin, lemon balm to calm, or peppermint on a muggy hot day to refresh and cool. Refreshing light herbal tisanes (teas) of lavender, chamomile, or calendula flowers are all suitable for cleansing a diaper rash; a nice, short dose of sunlight may help as well. Follow up with a light coating of an infusion of calendula flower oil.

BASIC HERBAL TISANE

1 teaspoon of selected fresh or dry herbs
1 cup boiling water

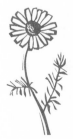

Place the herbs in a cup or teapot. Pour the hot boiling water over the herbs; cover, and let steep 5 to 15 minutes (depending on the herb). Strain and cool. Store a tisane in the refrigerator; if not used within 24 hours throw away or use leftover to water plants. The spent herbs can be added to compost. Chamomile can become bitter in just a few minutes so if you are making the tisane as a tea to drink only let steep for 2–3 minutes.

Check a reliable herbal (reference book) to determine the best preparation technique for the herb you're using.

Herbs for tisanes can be easily grown in your garden or in pots on a patio or deck. Dried herbs that can be used for tisanes are becoming much easier to find as people are becoming more aware of their potential to harmonize our lives. Herbal tea bags can be purchased in most groceries, health food stores, or farmer's markets in the fresh or dried form. Check around to locate your closest herbalist, or herb farm or shop.

HEATHFUL ROOM SCENTS

Undiluted essential oils are much too strong for young, sensitive skin. Never use a diffuser (which uses undiluted oil) in a baby's room. The pure essential oils are too concentrated, in my opinion, to be diffused into a baby's immature lungs.

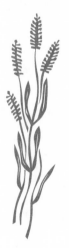

Simmer pot. A simmer pot, in which the oils are combined with water, can be used on a limited basis with a baby around. One or two drops of Roman chamomile or lavender essential oils added to a simmer pot of water may help calm the atmosphere; just be sure to place the simmer pot in a safe place where a child cannot touch it. A drop or two of eucalyptus can also be used to help clear the air in a sick baby's room.

Soap freshener. Adding a few drops of pure essential oils to soapy water makes a refreshing solution for cleaning and wiping down a child's room, including the crib frame, mattress cover, walls, and other washable surfaces. No more synthetic pine or lemon scents; you can get the real thing with essential oils! Lemon is refreshing, uplifting, and just smells clean. A quick wipe-down with eucalyptus can clear a room of a virus and disinfect. Lavender can be antiseptic and calming. Tea tree is considered a powerful household disinfectant and antiseptic.

Remember that the scents with which you surround your children will remain in their memories for a lifetime. Wouldn't you rather have those scents be natural and healthful? I also add essential oils to the liquid soaps I keep by the sink to disinfect and protect the hands as they're washing. Kids love to make lather and they do get their hands much cleaner (even if you're left with some extra soap suds to clean up — a good excuse to clean the sink!). Lemon, lavender, eucalyptus, tea tree, rose geranium, or bergamot oils all work well for this purpose.

Keep a natural bristle nail brush in a dish with interesting hand-made soaps near the sink. The brushing invigorates the nails and stimulates circulation.

Safety tips. Some general guidelines when blending pure essential oils for children include:

1. **Dilute, dilute, dilute!** When adding pure essential oils to anything that may come into direct contact with the skin, hands, or eyes always dilute them in a base. Base oils such as sweet almond, grapeseed, calendula-infused or jojoba oil work well for massage or skin care. Milk or cream are great bases for bath oils (or goat's milk for those allergic to cows); powdered milk also works well. Liquid castile soap is a good base for a shower.

2. **Shake or mix well!** Essential oils vary in viscousness and weight. Some oils, such as sandalwood, patchouli, and vanilla oleoresin, may drop to the bottom of a bottle of base oil of sweet almond, while other oils, such as lavender, frankincense, and Roman chamomile, spiral dance down the center of the bottle slowly. This is why a fragrance containing deep oils that sink may be called heavy while one with citrus oils that float is called light.

3. **Keep out of the reach of children.** Do not let a child handle pure essential oils. Keep children's contact with properly diluted oils to a minimum.

WARNING: KEEP DIFFUSERS AWAY FROM CHILDREN

If using a diffuser around children or pets please devise a safe place to put it, such as a special shelf mounted in a childproof place. I've heard too many stories about the dangers of leaving diffusers within reach of children. In one case history I was consulted about, a two-year-old drank essential oil from a diffuser left unattended in an older sibling's room for just a few minutes. A diffuser is glass, electrical, and full of powerful substances: pure, undiluted essential oils.

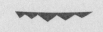

Product Tip
AROMATHERAPY FOR KIDS

When looking for aromatherapy products to benefit your whole family, become an avid label reader and learn to recognize good ingredients. Avoid any products with additives, extenders, synthetic ingredients, or a non-mineral oil base. Look for companies that will stand behind their products and ingredients. Search out the best, or, if you're so inclined, try making your own.

Aromatherapy for Kids (see resource list) is one company offering good quality products with such names as Lavender Lullaby Bubblebath, Lavender Lullaby Rub, Happy Bath, Happy Rub, and Ah-choo-lyptus Rub. They've got a great line for Mom and Dad too, including Rosebud Rub, Rockabye Mama Bath, Rockabye Mama Rub, Belly Butter, and Quiet Herbal Soak.

They also have a pure essential oil blend called Mother & Child created especially to calm and soothe the delicate harmony of Mom and baby, both physically and emotionally. This undiluted blend includes lavender, chamomile, fennel, and orange. To use, you simply add 6 drops to a tub of warm water for either your baby or yourself, or to a simmer pot with water kept near your favorite chair or bedside to use while you're nursing. A Mother & Child Massage Oil is also in a base of coconut oil. *Note:* I recommend caution when using anything containing fennel essential oil; while it's okay in a blend, fennel is rarely used alone.

Star Power Essentials (see resource list) is another maker of aromatherapy products for babies and mothers from oils that are obtained from plants that are either wildcrafted (gathered in the wild) or organically grown on small European farms. They produce an essential oil blend formulated to ease digestive upset, sedate nervous tension, promote lactation, and lift the spirits for new mothers.

NATURAL ROOM DISINFECTANT

6 drops of pure essential oil (lavender, lemon, eucalyptus, or tea tree)

2 gallons of soapy water (Castile or oil-based soaps work well)

Add essential oil to soapy water and mix well. Use a sponge or wet cloth to clean and disinfect the walls, furniture, and other exposed surfaces of your child's room.

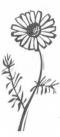

ALL-ROUND ESSENTIAL OIL BLEND

5 drops (or parts) lavender essential oil

5 drops (or parts) Roman Chamomile oil

1–2 drops (or parts) rose otto, optional (due to expense)

Combine oils in a small (4 ml) dark glass bottle and label well.

Massage oil: make a 1 percent dilution in almond oil.

Light room diffuser: add 2 to 3 drops to a simmer pot of water.

Occasional fragrant bath: dilute 2 to 3 drops in oil or milk and add to bathwater.

Aromatic water: add 1 drop to an 4 oz/118 ml spray bottle of spring water.

AROMATIC BABY BATHS

Bathing a baby or young child can be a special time for you both. I used to bathe Christina just before her nap. This relaxed her quite nicely. Some children may be stimulated by bathing. Observe your little one and decide what time is best for her.

A Shared Mother-Baby Bath

When Christina was an infant, I often bathed with her on my lap, and then called for Dad to come and wrap her up to cuddle before her nap. This would allow me a few extras moments to soak and relax. These shared baths helped engender in her a sense of trust and security in association with bathing. Some-times, I would wrap her in a hooded towel afterward and nurse her off to a nap; often I would rest, too.

Use 1 or 2 drops of lavender or chamomile pure essential oil to enhance the relaxing qualities of a baby's bath. Water should be warm, that is neither too hot nor too cool. Make sure any pure essential oils are well dispersed in the water so that baby doesn't get any on her hands or in the eyes or mouth. Diluting the essential oils first in milk, cream, or base oil will help assure that the baby won't get undiluted pure essential oils on the fingers and then in the mouth or eyes.

In the heat of summer, just 1 drop of peppermint oil well distributed in the water can be refreshing and cool-ing for you both. A sponge bath with some mild peppermint or spearmint herb tea is also a great sum-mer cool-down for little ones and big ones alike. After the bath,

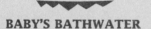

BABY'S BATHWATER

Some water contains high chemical and nitrite levels that can be dangerous to infants. Have your water tested before giving it to your baby, or bathing him in it. If you find high levels of chemicals in your water, you may want to look into water filters, which can help ensure better water quality.

Water temperature is also of the utmost importance. Floating thermometers are available that can assure you that the water is just the right temperature for your child.

a massage with an essential oil blend, plain sweet almond oil, or calendula flower oil (Weleda makes a good one) is a nice addition to the bathing ritual for you and baby.

As Christina got older, I took her in the shower with me and taught her not to be afraid of that method of cleaning up either. I also would sit her on the side of the tub to clean up messy little feet.

HERBAL BATH BAG FOR BABY

2 tablespoons fresh or dried mild herbs (see below)

Herbs for Baby's Bath:
Chamomile
Lavender
Lemon balm
Peppermint
Spearmint

Put the herbs into a cloth bag or an odd sock and tie a knot in the top. Toss this into a baby tub containing warm water and it will act like a very large tea bag. After bathing your baby (you don't have to remove the bag first), put the spent herbs into the compost pile or use to mulch your houseplants or outdoor container plants.

Always be aware of safety when bathing a baby: Keep objects out of reach of small hands, make sure water is not too hot, and exercise special caution when bathing baby in a slippery tub.

Here's a simple way to introduce fresh or dried herbs into your baby's care. Always attempt to buy the freshest ingredients available for your natural homemade products, or grow them yourself (see chapter 4).

EXTEND THE OLFACTORY TIE

If you used a particular blend of pure essential oils during pregnancy, you can extend the olfactory tie between you and your baby by adding the same blend to baby's bath. Add just 1 or 2 drops of the essential oil blend, diluted first in milk or cream, and mix well with a tub of warm water for baby's bath. Don't, however, use the same blend you may have used during labor. Odors evoke memories, and the birth process is probably not an experience you or your baby want to recall too vividly.

Bath Massage

A simple massage may be employed to wash a little one. The hands are a great tool; gentle, lightly pressured strokes help make a baby feel safe and comfortable in water. It can be fun and relaxing for adults, too. The water allows your hands to glide over his or her small frame without added oils or creams.

Try using a mild calendula soap or BASIS TM soap (available at any pharmacy). For more detailed instructions on massage techniques and massage oil recipes, see *Aromatherapy For Mother & Baby* by Allison England (see reading list). She also offers guidelines for which essential oils are safe to use in pregnancy and for baby.

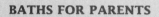

BATHS FOR PARENTS

Don't forget that mom and dad can benefit greatly from a special bath, as well — without baby! For an intoxicating, sensual, delightful adventure, add 1 or 2 drops each of ylang-ylang, patchouli, sandalwood, rose absolute, jasmine absolute, or vanilla oleoresin pure essential oil to your bathwater. A follow-up massage for each of you will go a long way toward reducing and releasing the stresses of parenthood!

CARING FOR NEW HAIR

Some babies are born with little hair, some with lots! Christina had long, thick, dark hair upon birth and it could be brushed shortly after. If your baby doesn't have much hair, a simple rinsing of the head with a wet washcloth will often suffice, but if he or she has a lot of hair, be prepared for more frequent washings.

The hair-washing experience can be a time of bonding and sharing for you and your baby.When I washed Christina's hair, I made it a pleasure for her by holding her securely with my arm underneath her back over a baby bath or the sink, and leaning her back over my arm while rinsing her hair with a small plastic cup. I gently massaged her head as I washed, speaking softly to her the whole time. A towel with a small triangular cap sewn into one end makes a great after-washing wrap. After the bath is a nice time to relax, nurse, cuddle, and even take a short nap if you both feel so inclined.

Shampoo

Never use harsh shampoos, soaps, bubble baths, or heavily scented synthetic products on baby — or on yourself, for that matter. Read the label of everything you buy and ask questions. Try to find products with the least number of ingredients with names that are hard to pronounce; avoid products whose contents are a mystery.

It's a good idea to keep a very mild shampoo or liquid castle soap near enough to the bath area that you can reach it with one hand, a top you can flip open with just one hand is great. For baby, Dr. Bronner's Castile Soap may also be used as a shampoo. It is mild, gentle, and basically unscented. If you want to rinse with a final herbal tisane of rosemary, or chamomile, keep that handy and properly cooled nearby.

Use only a drop or two of any shampoo on a baby's head. Less is best. Most shampoos and conditioners are very thick, and the bottles have large holes in the top so a lot comes out at a time. You don't need much. I suggest diluting all shampoos, conditioners, dish, laundry, and liquid soap with plain water before using on either yourself or your baby. I prefer to add pure essential oils to a base liquid soap to make hand and shower soaps.

A nice essential oil-enriched shampoo for both baby and mom is 2 drops of sandalwood, lavender, rose otto or Roman chamomile pure essential oil added to 1 tablespoon mild baby or jojoba shampoo. Use only a few drops of the shampoo, keep it well-labeled, shake well before use, and keep out of the eyes. Once again, do not use essential oil blends on a baby younger than three months. An infusion of 1 tablespoon dried chamomile, rosemary, nettle, calendula, or lavender herb made with one cup of water and then

BATHING BY CANDLELIGHT

A bath by candlelight is nice for a baby. Just be sure the candle is placed well away from baby's reach. The dark room and warm water may remind her of the womb. I suggest using beeswax candles when they are available; they have a wonderful natural scent. Don't use synthetically scented candles at all. A small oil lamp or a simmer pot with a candle (and water combined a few drops of a mild, pure essential oil in it) are also good options. Always use caution with candles around little ones.

added to a shampoo base also works well. This cool infusion may be used as a rinse after shampooing too. Use all of this at one shampooing.

Don't forget to enjoy the aromatic pleasures of shampoo enhanced with essential oils on your own hair, as well. I wore my long hair up when Christina was little, since having her little hands entangled in it was no fun. After washing, I would put it on top of my head in a hair tie while still damp, then roll it close to my head with my fingers and pin it in place with bobby pins. When I took it down in the evening, my hair was softly curled and carried the lovely smell of the herbs and pure essential oils I had used to cleanse and condition it. It swirled about my face in a redolent cloud as I brushed it out before bed.

Brushing

A soft brushing nicely stimulates the scalp. A soft, natural-bristle brush is best. You may also want to use small comb at times.

Conditioning

If you want to give your baby's hair a gentle conditioning treatment, I recommend using 2 tablespoons of a calendula-infused oil about once a month. (Weleda make a good one; see resource list.) For a baby older than three months, you can use a combination of 2 tablespoons of jojoba oil and 1 drop of tea tree or lavender essential oil, applied once a month. Do not, however, use any essential oils on a baby younger than three months.

Cradle Cap

Cradle cap is a crusty secretion that forms on babies' heads. Softening this with a calendula-infused oil, shampooing with a mild jojoba or castile-based shampoo, and then combing it out with a fine tooth comb is effective. For babies older than three months, try using a combination of 1 drop of sandalwood essential oil added to 1 teaspoon of a base oil such as sweet almond or jojoba. This can also be lightly massaged into the hair and scalp before shampooing.

Tub Cleaner

When you think about what goes into your baby's (and your) baths, don't forget the tub cleaner. Borax, sea salt, baking soda all make good natural tub cleaners, but *don't* use vinegar at the same time! Just as you discovered in the volcano experiment in grade school, combining vinegar with any of these bleach-con-taining products causes a chemical reaction (making it bubble up and overflow like lava) and produces toxic gases. Vinegar makes an excellent additive to a soak water for clothes, dishes, or diapers. Borax or baking soda can be used, but don't mix either one with vinegar.

FRESHENING DIAPERS AND CLOTHING NATURALLY

Cloth diapers are economical, better for baby, ecological, and comfortable. The cost is usually comparable to that of disposables, and you don't have to throw them away, so they can be used for another child. There are a number of companies offering cloth diapers (see resource list).

Diapering wisdom in the 1990s says forget pins and plastic pants. Velcro, diaper covers, and all-in-one diapers make cloth diapers the convenient and economical choice for parents today.

BASIC DIAPER SOAK

½ cup herbal vinegar
or
3 to 5 drops lemon, lavender, or tea tree pure essential oil

Add herbal vinegar or essential oil to a pail of diaper soak water. *Remember:* Do **not** add bleach to vinegar-soaked diapers in the wash.

Washing Diapers and Clothing

While shopping recently, I took an informal poll of mothers who were buying a specific laundry detergent especially targeted to wash baby clothes and diapers to determine why they chose that brand. The numbers were pretty evenly split. The loyalty factor was often to a brand used by someone else and recommended rather than to product performance. Allergic reactions were a factor, as was price. I'd opt for a detergent with the least perfume and dyes. Just because there is a picture of a baby on the box, that product is not necessarily any better for use on babies.

Most detergents have a toll-free consumer information number listed on their boxes; Call them and ask precisely why their product is better or even safe for your child. *The Natural Nursery* (see reading list) has a good section on commercial products and their ingredients, as well as their properties.

Check your local health food stores for laundry products that rely less on potentially toxic chemicals to cleanse. Baby soaps, shampoos, creams, oils, detergents, and powders can contain undesirable ingredients. They may contain preservatives, colorants, synthetic scents, emulsifiers, and other ingredients that extend shelf life, but don't do anything for your

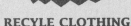

RECYCLE CLOTHING

Recycle children's clothing whenever possible. Quality clothing always outlasts babies, although it may not always survive the wear and tear from older kids. Go to resale shops, garage sales, and Goodwill stores. Churches often have recycled clothing programs or regular rummage sales. Exchange with friends and neighbors who have children in between your children's ages or solicit hand-me-downs from familes you know with older children. Passing outgrown clothing, maternity clothes, and baby equipment on to others you know is a great way to build community as well.

child's. Buyer beware, buyer be educated. Finding a mild natural detergent product to wash diapers also may help keep rashes and bad odors at bay.

Line-dry clothes and diapers whenever possible. Line-dried sheets and an aromatherapy bath are two of life's luxuries that I provide as often as possible for myself and for Christina. Right now, in late May, my bedroom has been thoroughly cleaned; fresh line-dried sheets, blankets, and pillows are on my bed; and the room is sweetly scented from jars filled with lily-of-the-valley, lilacs in five shades and scents, and violets from the gardens. When I sleep on these nights I feel at peace with the world. It is simple, inexpensive, and so special.

Selecting Clothing and Bedding

Product Tip
ORGANIC BEDDING AND CLOTHING

Earth Baby Inc. of Atlanta, Georgia (see resource list), offers alternatives to the usual baby stuff available to the public. Co-owners Mia Om and Reed Ricker were inspired by daughter Ko to find the products they wanted for her well-being. Their line of goods includes clothing from organic cotton — that is, grown without the use of synthetic fertilizers, herbicides, or pesticides. Their organic cotton goods are processed without bleach, formaldehyde, resins, or other chemical finishes. Only natural dyes are employed, which is healthier both for the farmworkers who labor to produce the raw materials needed and the babies who wear the fabric. In their Atlanta store, they also offer washable organic terry toys, children's furniture, storybooks with environmental themes, books for parents, and herbal and aromatherapy lines for parents and children.

Organic right down to the very clothes you put on your back, on your little one's tender young body? No synthetic fibers loaded with various chemicals? This sounds good to me. I recall opening clothes or bedding for my baby and knowing that the scent meant toxic chemicals had been used in their production and/or packaging. Materials are often treated with chemicals for any number of reasons, including as flame retardants, stain repellents, and for wrinkle resistance. I usually had to wash "new" things more than once to remove the store-bought scent. Comforters, blankets, sheets, pillows, bumper pads, and mattresses may also be treated.

Consider, too, what bedding and toys are stuffed with. I have always laughed at the tags that are meant to inform you of this. They used to say, *do not remove under penalty of law* or something similar to this. Now I believe the message is: The material content of the product is important for you to know about. The truth is, supplies and furniture we buy for our children are probably as toxic as any we buy for adults.

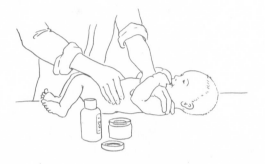

BABY CREAM, BALM, TINCTURES, AND POWDER

Of course, we would all like to make everything for baby as fresh and as pure as possible, which often means homemade. This isn't always possible and sometimes not at all practical. There are good suppliers of ready-made products available to you through local health food stores, and by mail order. Look for products with the simplest and most natural ingredients. Become familiar with natural ingredients. Invest in a good herbal cosmetics book such as Dorie Byers's *Natural Body Basics: Making Your Own Cosmetics* (see reading list) to introduce you to the ingredients and processes that fine natural products contain.

What to Look For

Look for balms and creams made with beeswax, pure base oils, and the best herbs and essential oils. While balm is very thick and meant to protect the skin, cream is less thick and formulated to penetrate the skin. Balms (also called salves) work best for healing burns, cuts, scrapes, diaper rash, skin

HERBAL BABY BALM

Base:

1 cup sweet almond oil

Herbs:

3 tablespoons dried lavender flowers

1 tablespoon dried calendula petals

1 tablespoon dried rose petals

1 teaspoon dried chamomile flowers

Emollients (to soften and soothe):

2 tablespoons vitamin E oil (10,000 international units)

1½ teaspoons jojoba oil

4 drops of either rose, Roman chamomile, or lavender essential oil

Emulsifier:

5 tablespoons beeswax

Yield:

Approximately 10 ounces (296 ml)

Grind the herbs into a powder using a clean coffee grinder, blender, or a mortar and pestle. Warm the base oil in the top of a double boiler pot; add the powdered herbs and cook over medium heat for 30 minutes to 1 hour to allow the healing properties of the herbs to be fully released in the oil.

Place the emollients in a stainless steel or glass bowl. Place a paper coffee filter inside a wire strainer, hold over the bowl, and pour the warm herb and base oil mixture through the strainer into the bowl. Gently apply pressure to the coffee filter to squeeze out most of the oil, being careful not to break it or spill any of the herbs.

Melt the beeswax in the top of a double boiler; add slowly to the oil and herb mixture while whisking with a Fresh whisk or egg beater. Continue whisking until the mixture is thick and creamy.

Sterilize several 2- to 4-ounce jars (jelly or baby-food jars work well) in freshly boiled water, so you have enough to hold approximately 10 ounces of finished balm. Fill each jar with balm, screw on the lid, and wipe off the jar. Label. If you plan to store balm for 3 months or more, refrigerate.

This recipe was developed by George Vutetakis of Inn Season Cafe in Royal Oak, Michigan. A balm is a fragrant ointment or aromatic oil that is healing, soothing, or helps mitigate pain or mental distress. It can be used to protect baby's bottom from getting chapped or dry, and is great for softening dry skin spots on little hands or feet.

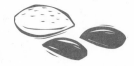

infections, and a host of other external complaints. I keep jars of balm close at hand in the kitchen, garage, workshop, by the woodstove, fireplace, and in the medicine chest. Ointments are similar to balms, but they contain less beeswax, making for a softer product. These both penetrate and protect the skin.

A great sourcebook of methods for making herbal baby products at home is *Natural Healing for Babies and Children* by Aviva Jill Romm (see reading list). She also includes some of the best advice on home healing I have ever seen. This book would make an excellent shower gift combined with a selection of dried herbs, herb plants, and/or some of the basic ingredients a mom could use to create some herbal allies before baby is born.

Gary's Baby Balm Recipes

Gary L. Wanttaja of Nature's Products in Detroit, Michigan makes and sells his own herbal products. He generously shared these wonderful smelling and luxuriously nourishing balm recipes. He notes that in naming the recipes, he doesn't intend to limit their uses, which are many. Any of these balms could be used for chapped skin, lip balm, skin care, after-bath balm, belly balm, or baby's bottom balm. Cocoa butter is great for preventing stretch marks, and can also be used for dry, sore feet. As you become familiar with each ingredient, you'll learn the many ways it can be used.

These recipes are all very mild and are particularly effective because they are freshly made. Gary recommends always using the best and freshest ingredients available. You may find that you will want to vary the proportions of ingredients slightly depending on the time of year and temperature when you are making the recipe, and your personal taste.

Once you've discovered how useful and versatile these recipes are, you'll want to be sure to have a jar of each on hand. Keep one in the diaper bag, one in your purse, one in the bathroom, and one in the car, and discover how handy these balms can be. Just be sure to keep them out of the reach of children, and away from extreme heat or cold (which will change their consistency).

CALENDULA CREAM

4 ounces shea butter

2 tablespoons dried (or fresh) calendula flowers

800 international units vitamin E oil

3 drops rose otto essential oil

30 drops lavender essential oil

Small, wide-mouthed glass jar (recycled baby-food jars work well)

10 drops tincture of benzoin, optional (as a natural preservative)

Melt the shea butter in the top of a double boiler; add the calendula flowers and heat over medium heat for 30 to 40 minutes, stirring occasionally. Pour mixture through a strainer to remove the calendula flowers. Add the essential oils and the vitamin E oil. Pour into jar (best if the cream fills the jar); once mixture is cool, close with lid. Label the jar.

Yield: Approximately 4 ounces (118 ml)

SKIN PROTECTING BALM

4 ounces shea butter

2 tablespoons jojoba oil

2 tablespoons (⅔ ounce) beeswax

16 drops rose geranium essential oil

6 drops Roman chamomile essential oil

800 international units vitamin E oil

10 drops tincture of benzoin, optional (as a natural preservative)

Small, wide-mouthed glass jar

Melt shea butter and beeswax in the top of a double boiler. Add remaining ingredients. Allow to cool, then pour into jar and close tightly. Label the jar.

Yield: Approximately 6 ounces (177 ml)

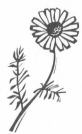

BEYOND-THE-BATH BALM

4 ounces shea butter
1 tablespoon beeswax
1 tablespoon apricot kernel oil
1 tablespoon avocado oil
800 international units
    vitamin E oil
20 drops sandalwood
    essential oil
10 drops tincture of benzoin,
    optional (as a natural
    preservative)
Small, wide-mouthed glass jar

Melt shea butter in top of double boiler. Add remaining ingredients and mix well. Allow to cool, then pour into jar and close tightly. Label the jar.

Yield: Approximately 5½ ounces (173 ml)

BOSOM, BELLY, AND BOTTOM BUTTER

3 ounces shea butter
1 tablespoon cocoa butter
1 tablespoon beeswax
30 drops lavender essential oil
8 drops rosewood essential oil
800 international units
    vitamin E oil
10 drops tincture of benzoin,
    optional (as a natural
    preservative)
Small, wide-mouthed glass jar

Melt shea butter in top of double boiler. Add remaining ingredients and mix well. Allow to cool, then pour into jar and close tightly. Label the jar.

Yield: Approximately 4½ ounces (133 ml)

BLUE MOON BALM

4 ounces shea butter
1 tablespoon beeswax
1 tablespoon rosehip seed oil
5 drops yarrow oil
10 drops sandalwood
    essential oil
800 international units
    vitamin E oil
10 drops tincture of benzoin
Small, wide-mouthed glass jar

Melt shea butter in the top of a double boiler. Add remaining ingredients and mix well. Allow to cool, then pour into a jar and close tightly. *Note:* Tincture of benzoin is essential in this recipe because rosehip seed oil sometimes has a very short shelf life. Label the jar.

Yield: Approximately 5 ounces (158 ml)

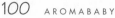

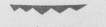

Product Tip
BABY CREAMS, SALVES, AND GELS

Country Comfort's Baby Cream is formulated to protect delicate skin, and to be applied between diaper changes. This cream combines pure beeswax, lanolin (check for allergies), pure oils of safflower, sweet almond, avocado, and apricot, with fresh herbal extracts of chamomile, chickweed, comfrey, calendula, golden seal, St.-John's-wort, myrrh gum, and aloe vera. It also contains vitamins and pure wintergreen oil. *Note:* Wintergreen oil is *not* recommended for general use. It can only be used in very small proportions, as it is in this cream. Never use wintergreen oil for aromatherapy.

Weleda, Inc. (see resource list) makes an incredible Calendula Baby Cream that contains pure essential oils of rose, bergamot, and rose geranium. It also contains beeswax, calendula extract, and peanut oil (avoid when your baby has allergies). This cream forms a protective layer that soothes baby's tender skin. It is used as a moisture shield. This cream smells absolutely wonderful. Weleda also carries a Medicated Baby Cream with zinc oxide.

Calendula Gel, made by Boericke & Tafel, Inc. (see resource list), is valuable when dealing with irritated skin, scrapes, sunburn, eczema, and rough, chapped hands. Gels are cool, soothing, nongreasy, easy to carry and use, and great for kids.

The recipe for Country Comfort's (see resource list) Pure Herbal Salve is based on an early-16th-century herbal. (I have always said the farther you look back, the farther ahead you can see!) It contains a harmonious blend of herbs, pure vegetable oils, vitamins E, A, and D, and pure beeswax. They are designed to protect the skin and comfort while the body performs its healing functions.

Country Comfort also makes Golden Seal–Myrrh Savvy, an all-purpose blend for infections, scrapes, and cuts, and Comfrey–Aloe Vera Herbal Savvy, a powerful combination of very gentle herbs for sunburn, burns, chapped skin, and diaper rash. Their Baby Oil is composed of the finest safflower, sweet almond, jojoba, and olive oils, along with rosemary and vitamin E. Its uses include moisturizing and cleansing delicate skin. Apply it with cotton to prevent chafing for dryness, cradle cap, and to safely clean baby's outer ears, nose, and navel. This oil is made to be packaged within 24 hours of blending to ensure freshness.

Tinctures

A tincture is an alcoholic herbal preparation. The alcohol draws the herb's benefits into it. It can then be diluted and applied directly to the skin to help heal scrapes and bruises on older children.

Tinctures are fairly easy to make. I keep busy making them in the summer so that my household will have plenty to see us through the winter. You can use dried herbs if necessary, but I much prefer fresh — I get a more potent product using the lovely calendula flowers newly cut from the backyard herb garden. Moreover, they make beautiful colorful decorations while they steep!

I also annually make echinacea, myrrh, and St. John's wort tincture and motherwort tincture for our use. Echinacea is an excellent immune system stimulant. Myrrh is antiseptic and astringent. St.-John's-wort is healing to the nerves. Tinctures can also be added to creams, salves, and ointments to extend their shelf life and enhance their healing abilities.

I also make a wonderful skin-care oil from St.-John's-wort. The bright yellow flower turns the oil base red. If you squeeze an unopened flower of St.-John's-wort between your fingers, it

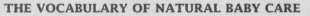

THE VOCABULARY OF NATURAL BABY CARE

Remember, with children some things take "tincture of time." I first heard this from a doctor when Christina was 15 and quite sick with strep throat. Assuming the doctor meant tincture of *thyme*, I promptly agreed that thyme was indeed antiseptic and that I had included a small amount of the pure essential oil in a simmer pot to ease congestion, although I had not thought of using it in tincture form. I was so glad to hear an M.D. give this type of advice. A very bewildered doctor looked at me as though I was from Mars. "I meant this may take a while to heal," she said. She had no idea what tincture of thyme may be. She told me what she'd said was something she had learned in medical school.

will stain them a purple-red. Kids think it's cool to see and do. St.-John's-wort is the source of the homeopathic remedy Hypericum, the "stepped-on-a-nail remedy." This is included in most standard kits for kids; that makes at least three useful household products from one herb. Both are used to heal nerve injury and to speed the healing of wounds or bites. It's especially helpful after a bump on the head or before surgery. Tincture, homeopathic remedy, and skin care oil: All come from one beautiful plant. I allow St.-John's-wort to grow at will in my gardens.

CALENDULA TINCTURE

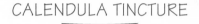

4 handfuls of fresh flowers
1-quart clean glass jar

Put the herbs in the glass jar. Fill jar to top with grain alcohol. Screw on top and let steep for 2 to 4 weeks (from the new moon to the full moon). Strain the alcohol through a coffee filter to get the tincture. Pour strained tincture into a dark glass bottle and seal well.

To use, dilute 1 part tincture in 10 parts fresh water or witch hazel. Apply directly to scrapes, rashes, stings, and to clean any skin problems. You can also put this mixture in a small spray bottle, to be used in a few days because it has no preservatives. To disinfect on the spot I have used it undiluted. It stings, but it works. This is actually an herbal remedy as much as a homeopathic one.

Yield: 1 quart

Calendula is effective for irritations and inflammations, relieving itching and stinging. It is antiseptic, and soothing for rashes, cuts, scrapes, diaper rash, and burns. It is an excellent addition to beauty products such as creams, facial steams, or hair rinses. Its lovely yellow or orange flowers are a beautiful accent for your garden, as well.

Powdering Baby

Always exercise caution when using powder; talc can be harm-ful. Use only small amounts, if necessary, and avoid inhalation by either yourself or your baby. Apply powder to your hand and then to baby.

BASIC BABY POWDER

3 ounces kaolin clay
½ teaspoon myrrh powder
3 drops rose, lavender, or
   Roman chamomile
   essential oil

Combine all ingredients in a small jar or bottle and mix well. Use sparingly by applying powder first to your hand and then to baby.

Yield: Approximately 3 ounces (79 ml)

Product tip
BABY POWDER

Country Comfort (see resource list) makes a baby powder that is very absorbent because it has a base of pure mineral clay. The gentle healing properties of five herbal powders — arrowroot, comfrey, slippery elm, gold-enseal, and aloe vera — are combined with the subtle scents of pure orange and lavender oils. These pure ingredients absorb moisture that can cause irritation and chafing. These powders can be used after the bath or diaper changes to soothe and protect delicate skin.

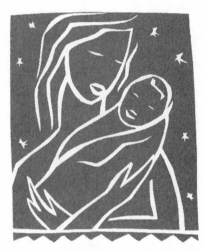

Natural Ways
To Raise A
Happy, Healthy,
Growing Baby

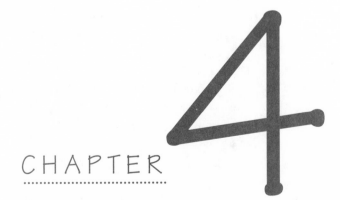

CHAPTER

An important part of raising a baby naturally is to put some thought and your heart into learning about techniques, practices, and events that will bring you closer and help promote growth and good health for all of you. Once you start exploring, you may be surprised at how many things you can do yourself, at home, to help soothe, calm, and strengthen your baby. Look beyond the conventional and you'll find all kinds of ideas.

What goes into your baby's body is just as important as what goes on your baby's body. While you should always seek the advice of your medical professional before attempting to treat any illness or condition your baby suffers from, there are things you can do to help prevent illness, from making sure your baby gets enough of your loving touch through nurturing and massage, to carefully controlling what your baby eats, to using homeopathic remedies to help prevent illness.

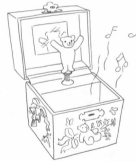

SOOTHING A BABY TO SLEEP

My, how the words "baby go to sleep" ring clear in the minds of many parents who were a few hours shy of much-needed rest after trying to comfort an infant. Advice like "Let them cry it out" is fine from people who don't have to be there to witness your little one's distress or discomfort, whatever the cause. A babe's cry is meant to irritate us. It is a distress signal. Something is wrong and making him uncomfortable, so his cry makes you, or any other caregiver, uncomfortable. That's how nature designed it.

Along with the tapes, Woodford includes some tips for helping babies sleep. Here are a few of his tips for an easier bedtime:

◆ Create a regular routine for your child.
◆ Complete final steps of unwinding for bedtime in the room where the child sleeps.
◆ The child needs to fall asleep where she will wake up.
◆ If you allow a baby always to fall asleep on the couch or your lap or while being rocked, cuddled, or fed, that is surely where the baby will want to continue to fall asleep.

- After calming a child, put her in her own bed and allow her to calm herself further to sleep. When she awakens in the night, she will have developed the ability to calm herself to some degree on her own.
- The last awake impression for a child should be in her own room, in her own bed.

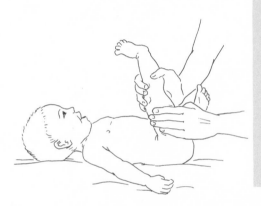

INFANT MASSAGE

Touch is one of the most important gifts and healing remedies we can give or receive. In today's society, we are often touch-deprived. Massage can be a wonderful way to foster relaxation, nurturing, and sharing for you and your child. For both parents, massage is a wonderful way to get to know your baby.

As a parent or caregiver, you can enhance a relationship through therapeutic touch. My relationship with my own daughter benefits from massage therapy to this day, when she is 16 years old. When she comes in tired from work she will ask me to massage her feet. This is a practice I have employed with her since she was a baby. She is always ready for a full body massage from a visiting massage therapist, and enjoys an occasional office appointment. She views this as the treat that it truly is — we both deeply appreciate massage.

You need not take a massage course (although you may certainly want to consider one). All you need is the desire to soothe a baby or child and a gentle hand. There are many good books available on massage therapy that enable you to learn in the privacy of your home. I'm always observant while a qualified massage therapist works, to glean some of her techniques.

For a tiny baby, even the stroking of his body lightly with a finger is stimulating enough to let him know you are there and care. We have become such a touch-phobic society that the safe, reassuring touch of a loving parent can be a haven in an often confusing and difficult world. Include your spouse in your massage therapy plans.

Benefits

The benefits of infant massage are rapidly becoming recognized, the most important benefit being the bonding that can occur between parent and child. Beyond the immediate physical benefits (see following list), there are also many psychological benefits to infant massage. Lack of touch stimulation for infants has been linked to problems later in life, ranging from hyperactivity to criminal behavior.

The various strokes and rhythms used in massage are not hard to grasp especially when one is filled with maternal or paternal love. Renee M. Gauthier, an infant massage expert who is nationally certified in therapeutic massage and bodywork and by the Academy of Certified Birth Educators (see resource list), conducts a complete prenatal and infant massage program called "Whole Mother/Nurtured Child" at Irenes Myomassology Institute in Southfield, Michigan.

Renee notes the following beneficial effects of massage on infant behavior and experience:

◆ Improved sleeping and calmer, deeper sleep
◆ More relaxed and aware in their space
◆ Improved sucking; helps the infant to gain weight and allows less air consumption which limits gas or abdominal discomfort
◆ Aids in joint movement which helps with crawling, standing, and walking

- Elimination of bodily wastes becomes easier
- Parents develop a deeper bond with their infant
- Cleanses the lymphatic system which helps the infant to stay healthier
- Stimulates growth hormones and endorphins, fostering faster growth and a happier baby
- Faster neurological growth
- Increased circulation which increases blood supply and nutrition to muscles
- Relief of congestion
- Relaxes muscle spasms and tension

Massage is also invaluable for children with special needs, such as cerebral palsy, deafness, or those born drug-addicted.

How to Begin

Renee Gauthier advises the best way to learn about infant massage is to contact a state licensed school and ask for a reference to a licensed and certified practitioner who teaches parents individually about this precious parenting skill. The International Myomassethics Federation, which licenses therapists, and instructors in prenatal and infant massage, is one group you can consult (see resource list). There are also a number of good books on this topic (see reading list).

If you want to hire a massage therapist to work on your child or yourself, interview him or her just as you would anyone else you would hire, especially someone coming into your home. Feel free to ask about professional training and accreditation. Do not accept a nonaccredited therapist. Touching you or your child's body is a very special job, one that requires someone with whom you are completely comfortable. As infant massage gains in popularity and training becomes more readily available, you should have no trouble in finding a qualified therapist.

Massage therapy is a respected profession and its benefits are far-reaching. Many classes and courses are now available on various massage techniques, ranging from community education classes to diploma courses that can run for months and turn out a professional massage therapist.

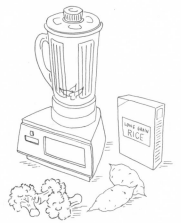

FEEDING BABY ORGANICALLY

Choosing when and what to feed your child is a serious and personal decision. I recall thoroughly rethinking my diet during pregnancy, lactation, and in the first young years of my child's life. My husband and stepson weren't as eager to change their diets, so providing good food wasn't always easy or appreciated. The naturally nutritious foods I prepared were referred to as "rabbit food" or "bird food" on more than one occasion. So don't be put off or be too disappointed if everyone in the family isn't as enthusiastic as you are to reap the benefits of a whole-foods or an organically grown diet. Assure them that you want the best for all members of the family. Instilling guilt isn't usually effective in helping people change their dietary habits. Instilling self-esteem would seem to be a much better method.

When we ingest healthy foods we feel good, or at the least better. We love it when one of our good habits or life practices comes back to us via our children, but boy, how we hate it when the negative ones do also. Convincing a family that natural, organically grown foods are the best may take some doing, but it's ultimately worth the effort. With small ones, you'll be providing the best beginning you can.

Introducing Foods to Baby

The introduction of foods varies with each child. Invest in a good book on baby nutrition, such as *The Baby Cookbook: A Complete Guide to Nutrition, Feeding, and Cooking for Babies Six Months to Two Years of Age* by Karin Knight, R.N. and Jeannie Lumley (see reading list). This book includes 200 recipes for nutritious family meals that babies and toddlers can share.

Check for any noticeable food allergies by introducing one food at a time, and keenly observe your child's reactions. (A reaction may be a rash, hives, cramps, headache, frequent urination, congestion, emotional acting out, red cheeks, stomachache, gas, diarrhea, constipation, or any other number of symptoms.) Keep a little notebook to record reactions and the offending foods. *Dr. Mandell's 5-Day Allergy Relief System* is an interesting book on the subject of food allergies (see reading list). Some common food allergens include wheat, corn, dairy products, food dyes, oats, nuts, shellfish, eggs, beef, chicken, chocolate, soy products, oranges, strawberries, coffee, tomatoes, and potatoes.

People may react to the pesticides and chemical fertilizers that are so often used in modern farming. Babies certainly don't need these in their delicate, young systems. In the name of cosmetically pleasing fruits and vegetables, we have given up quality and nutrition and introduced dangerous chemicals into our food chain as well. Fruits and vegetables that are imported are apt to contain chemicals; not all countries have restrictions on their use. Irradiation is also likely in many fruit and vegetables we buy today. Improper washing and peeling can increase the chances of ingesting pesticides, fumigants, fungicides, and chemical fertilizers.

Ollie and George Blezinski, whom I refer to as my godparents (because I'm convinced they were gifts from God to make my world a much better place), are the people most responsible for enlightening me to the benefits of organic farming and foods. Now in their 80s, they have much life experience and graciously share that knowledge with anyone willing to listen to their wonderful stories. They have farmed organically for many years — since long before it became popular. They believe that pesticides and chemical fertilizers have no place in farming. One look at their bright eyes, smiling faces, and kind demeanor

Product Tip
ORGANIC BABY FOOD

Earth's Best (see resource list) was the first "certified organically grown" baby food on the national market. They process their foods using only whole fruits, grains, and vegetables. No refined sugar, salt, fillers of any kind, or modified starches are added.

Earth's Best also produces a line of organic junior foods, the nation's only certified organic foods specifically designed to meet the nutritional needs of older infants. Their foods are available in supermarkets in selected cities, and in natural food stores across the country. The company also publishes a parenting newsletter.

will quickly and easily convince you that they have wonderful knowledge to share. There were days when they worked circles around me and still had energy and enthusiasm to create a gourmet meal.

Let us teach our children that there is a better way to garden, the natural way. My godparents are the proof.

The Benefits of Feeding Organically

Babies' small bodies are particularly vulnerable to the effects of pesticides. The brain and the immune system are immature in infants, and experience rapid growth. Infants and children in general receive greater exposure to pesticides in foods than do adults. For example, a non-nursing child may consume 16 times more apple juice than the average consumer, and fruit crops are

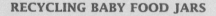

RECYCLING BABY FOOD JARS

If you or someone you know uses baby food that comes in a jar, be sure to recycle the jars. Here are a few ideas for their uses.

♦ Massage oils can be put up in these little glass jars. Although oils are best kept in dark-colored glass or plastic, baby-food jars are so small that the contents will be used quickly and won't oxidize from the light.

♦ Make an all-natural herbal potpourri from your garden. Punch holes in the jar lid so the scent is released into the room.

♦ Make bug jars to observe insects. I always had a rule that we could watch them for an hour and then we had to let them go.

♦ Use to store dried culinary herbs in a dark cool cupboard.

♦ Small amounts of leftovers fit nicely into baby-food jars. Remember to put baby's food in a bowl before you begin feeding her. Do not feed from the jar; the saliva can contaminate the food from the spoon. Resist the urge to have a taste and then give one to baby.

♦ Homemade salves and creams like these little storage jars. Always exercise caution with glass. Homemade labels will decorate them nicely. Include instructions as well as contents. (See recipes on pages 99–100.)

♦ Use as mini-greenhouses to cover and protect tender seedlings.

frequently sprayed with chemicals. "It is now widely suspected that the largest contribution to an individual's lifetime risk of cancer from pesticide residue occurs during childhood," says Lisa Bell of Earth's Best, Inc., a manufacturer of organic baby foods. These findings are backed up in a report entitled *Pesticides in Children's Food,* which says that "millions of children in the United States receive up to 35 percent of their entire lifetime dose of some carcinogenic pesticides by age five." Seventy pesticides have been pinpointed as causing cancer in laboratory animals (adequate data concerning the health effects of pesticides is not available, says Bell).

These findings are further supported by the Environmental Working Group (EWG). President Kenneth A. Cook reports some alarming statistics in the group's literature, titled Pesticides in Baby Food. According to laboratory tests commissioned by EWG, 16 pesticides were found in eight brand-name baby foods produced by three of the dominant baby-food makers in the market. Some babies get another dose of pesticides from drinking water, says Cook, or from bug sprays and weed killers used around the home. He elaborates on these disturbing results in his executive summary by saying that the Food and Drug Administration's standard pesticide analytical methods were used in discovering these findings. Further, he explains what should already be obvious to these baby-food manufacturers: that "infants and children are not little adults." He explains that their reactions to many drugs and toxins are different from adult responses, and most of the time they suffer serious injury to their health.

EWG's study reveals that fruits contain more pesticides than do vegetables, and at higher levels. Cook writes that five

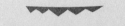

KEEPING YOUR CHILD'S DIET HEALTHY

Lisa Bell of Earth's Best Inc., a Boulder, Colorado, manufacturer of organic baby food, says these steps will help concerned parents ensure that their children's diets are healthy:

◆ Purchase foods that have been organically grown. These are easy to find at natural and whole food markets, and at a growing number of supermarkets. Ask your favorite grocers to carry more organic products.
◆ Never buy waxed produce.
◆ Peel all nonorganic fresh fruits and vegetables whenever possible.

different pesticides were found in pears; four in applesauce; and three in peaches, plums, and green beans. Iprodione (Rovral) is classified by the Environmental Protection Agency as a probable cause of cancer in humans. It was found only in peaches and plums, but more often than any other pesticide that was detected.

Buying Organically

If you aren't fortunate enough to have an Ollie and George who grow and share their organic produce, a local farmer's market, or an active food co-op, at least consider this: When shopping in grocery stores, try to stay in the perimeter of the store. Shop for 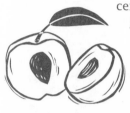 *live* foods: fresh produce, dairy products, meats, cheeses, and fruits. Most foods in the aisles are processed, that is, something is left out, or something is added in. In other words, not natural. What a scary concept, unnatural. Think about it when washing and preparing foods for yourself and the precious little ones you have been entrusted to care for. Encourage your local market to expand their organic foods section. Assure them that they will have your business if they provide the best for you and your family.

Organic gardening is gentle, self-paced, healthy, deeply satisfying, and environmentally friendly. Purchasing organically grown foods says yes, we support Mother Earth in all of her natural abundance. Remember her on Mother's Day . . . every day.

We will be fed better when we create the demand for more organically grown goods and are willing to pay the price to obtain them. The monetary price to achieve a healthier lifestyle is preferable to the price that is paid by poor nutrition, which is the decline of our health, body, mind, and spirit.

WHAT DOES "ORGANIC" MEAN?

The word "organic" describes the process by which a food has been prepared. "Organically grown" means that the food had been grown without the use of synthetic pesticides and fertilizers. Cover crops, natural fertilizers, and compost are used by organic farmers to build healthy soils to grow their produce in. Federal standards were established through the Organic Food Protection Act of 1990. The U.S. Department of Agriculture was scheduled to implement the act sometime in 1995, after which all organic foods on the market would be required to be certified as organically grown and processed. "Certified," in this case, would mean that the organic claim is verified by a qualified third party.

Try to be more aware of your daily diet. Think about what, how, and when you eat. Read labels, ask questions, take classes, join a food co-op, start a food co-op, wash your foods, and whenever possible, grow your own. Everything tastes so divine when it's perfectly in season.

Making Your Own Organic Baby Food

George Vutetakis, Chef and Proprietor of the Inn Season Café in Royal Oak, Michigan was generous enough to share some of his expertise on making healthful, appealing organic food for infants and small children. Following are his guidelines.

Use foods that are quality, fresh products. Organically grown, or at least pesticide-free, foods are best for ensuring that invisible or unknown ingredients are avoided in your child's diet.

Avoid spicy foods or strong spices. Food that is mild with a sweet (not sugary) flavor is preferable. Turmeric is a good, mild blood purifier when used in small amounts. Too much (spoonfuls) may cause anemia. Sweet spices like cinnamon, nutmeg, and coriander add to vitality. Fennel may aid digestion. Fresh mint is a digestive aid. Basil, oregano, and other Mediterranean herbs offer flavor and pizzazz to normally bland food.

TIPS FOR PROMOTING HEALTHY EATING

◆ Children of all ages love fun-shaped whole grain noodles as finger food. (They also love brown rice, but it is pretty messy.)

◆ For newly teething babies, try giving them either whole grain crackers or cold carrots.

◆ Try to avoid giving children large quantities of raisins and dried fruits — they promote tooth decay.

◆ Use rice, soy, or almond milks and cheese as your "dairy" of choice. Many children are lactose-intolerant. Also, cow's milk can contribute to a number of ailments from an upset stomach to an ear infection.

◆ Remember who the parent is! Young children can digest just about anything, so you can make decisions about what to feed them. I once had to remind a mother of this when she told me her daughter would eat nothing but Spaghetti-O's for a week. We set the example, so remember to eat your vegetables, chew your food well, say a prayer of gratitude, and make mealtime a family time (no TV please!).

Use dairy products lightly or avoid all together, if possible. If you must use them, yogurt (made with organic whole milk) in moderation is preferable. According to ancient East Indian traditions, whole milk contains a balance of lactates that allows for better digestion of the milk itself. Also, non-homogenized milk is better because homogenization scrambles the molecular structure of the milk which makes it more difficult to digest.

Look for local dairies that vat-pasteurize and pasture feed their herd. Most commercial milk is steam-pasteurized at high temperatures that destroy the good as well as the bad in milk. To keep profitable, many modern dairy farms feed their herds inside, not wasting time and energy on pasturing.

A positive alternative is goat's milk. It is closer to human milk and is excellent for children, especially those with a lactose intolerance. For information on goat's milk and to obtain fresh goat cheeses, Rivendell Meadows in Vermont is an excellent source of produce and information (see resource list). You might also consider rice, soy, or almond milks.

After your child cuts the first tooth, grains may be added to his diet. Make sure they are soft and mushy. Puree with vegetables such as carrots, yams, or squash. Cooked peas or other well-cooked legumes may be added to create a whole protein.

Basic Recipes

To supplement nursing or for new little eaters who have just been weaned, George suggested a variety of foods from organic lightly cooked greens to whole-grain porridge. "They have a fresh set of taste buds that will adapt to anything," he says. "A lot of sweetener isn't needed, especially no white refined sugar, which can weaken the immune system." The grains used in these recipes are usually available in bulk at natural food stores.

SWEET VEGETABLES

Squash, carrots, and sweet potatoes

Cook one or a mixture of the vegetables until they are soft. Serve in small chunks or mash first in a baby-food grinder.

ADVANCE PREPARATION TIPS FOR HOMEMADE BABY FOODS

George Vutetakis says that preparing healthy baby foods can be quite easy, even with a demanding child, as long as you do a little bit of advance planning, thinking, and preparation. Here are some suggestions for how to do it.

◆ Prepare a base of brown rice, millet, or quinoa (*keen-wah*, mother grain of the Andes). Make enough for a couple of days.

◆ Peel an avocado ahead of time and store it by rinsing it with cold water and wrapping it. Mash as needed.

◆ Prepare carrots or other vegetables in advance by placing in a casserole with a spritz of tamari (aged soy sauce), bay leaf, a cinnamon stick, and water to cover the bottom. Cover. Bake, airtight, for 45 minutes to an hour at 350°–400°F. When cool, remove bay leaf and cinnamon stick. This preparation process softens the carrots while preserving their nutrients.

◆ Prepare beans in advance by soaking overnight. The next day, drain beans and place in a large pot. Cover with fresh water, add a piece of kombu (a Japanese sea vegetable available at health food stores) to aid digestion, and boil until soft. Save some of the cooking water to use as stock in rice, baked vegetables, and soups. This contributes a small amount of protein to the diet.

MILLET AND SQUASH PORRIDGE

1 cup rinsed millet
½ cup cubed butternut
   squash
4 cups pure water
1 pinch sea salt

Combine the millet, squash, water, and salt in a saucepan and bring to a boil. Reduce heat and simmer for 20 to 25 minutes; do **not** stir as this will cause the millet to develop air pockets and stick to the pan. Remove from heat and mash in a baby-food grinder, adding a little organic tahini or rice syrup for additional calcium and sweetness, if desired.

Variations: In place of 1 cup millet, substitute a combination such as: ¾ cup millet and ¼ cup teff; ¾ millet and ¼ cup amaranth; or ½ cup millet and ½ cup brown rice.

QUINOA AND OAT FLAKES PORRIDGE

1½ cups pure water
A pinch of sea salt
¼ cup rinsed quinoa
¼ cup oat flakes

Combine the water and salt in a saucepan and bring to a boil. Add the grains, reduce heat, and simmer for 15 minutes, stirring occasionally.

BROWN RICE

2¼ cups water
½ teaspoon olive oil
¼ teaspoon sea salt
1 cup brown rice

Combine water, oil, and salt in a saucepan and bring to a boil. Add rice and return to boil. Cover pan, lower heat, and let simmer for 45 minutes. Turn off heat. Allow covered pan to sit for 10 minutes before serving.

COOKED GREENS

½ cup pure water
A pinch of sea salt
Organic kale, collard greens, or broccoli, rinsed with stems removed

Combine water and salt in a saucepan and bring to a boil. Add the greens and cover. Cook for 2–3 minutes, until soft but still bright green. Drain immediately so minerals are not lost in the water. Mash in a baby-food grinder.

These greens are very high in calcium.

FRUIT COMPOTE

½ cup organic apple juice
A pinch of sea salt
1 cup cubed organic apples or pears

Combine juice and salt in a saucepan and bring to a boil. Add the cubed fruit and cook until soft. Serve as is or mash. *Note:* Because different enzymes are needed to digest fruits as opposed to whole grains, do not combine whole grains and any kind of fruit. It can cause a very upset tummy.

PERSONAL TESTIMONY: GEORGE VUTETAKIS' APPROACH TO FEEDING CHILDREN

Whether your diet is macrobiotic, vegetarian, Pritikin, live foods, or meat and potatoes, balance, moderation, and understanding are essential. Diets that have been here for hundreds or thousands of years have a track record and are based on harmony with nature. If you have a distinct philosophy about maintaining a harmonious diet, raising a child within that framework works well. There are some difficulties: having to cook from scratch most, or all, of the time; finding traditional ingredients; how your child's diet may affect relationships with other children or families; and being able to provide nutritional variety in the diet (traditional vegetarian diets are based on grouping foods together rather than an entrée with a side dish).

My son has been raised as a lacto-vegetarian (vegetarian with milk products). Dietary health problems have not been an issue. He has stuck to being vegetarian of his own volition. He had some hard times at school, as kids can be unkind about anyone who is a little different. At one point, I had to package his lunch to look like what the other kids were eating. Now he is in a school where the majority of kids are familiar with a vegetarian diet. (In fact, many of them are vegetarians.)

Once you've decided to prepare healthier foods, some attitudes may need adjustment. The first is to remember that fresh foods and quality products are important. A lower price may reflect less healthfulness. Second, we can stuff many vitamins and foodstuffs with added nutrients into our bodies, but the body absorbs nutrients best when consumed in a natural state. Thus, avoid overcooked food. Steam vegetables, use the water, bake in sealed containers, and use fresh whenever possible.

Food allergies are unpleasant and may be difficult to ascertain. An allergist can help to determine what the specific problem foods are. One food group seems to affect allergies most: dairy products. You may have to reduce or eliminate milk and cheeses especially if the symptoms are sinus-oriented. This is corroborated by most ancient medical approaches as well as my own family's experience. If the allergies are to products like corn or wheat, read labels carefully, as many food bases use derivatives.

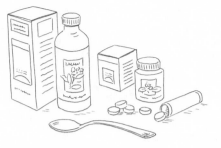

HERBAL REMEDIES FOR CHILDREN: A MEDICINAL APPROACH

It isn't likely that you'll have the time and herbs to manufacture your own medicinal products. Of course if you can, and it appeals to you, that's great, but if not, don't despair — many fine products are available commercially. There are strong restrictions imposed in the United States in regard to making medicinal claims; therefore, it is important that you be familiar with the benefits of various products when you order. Their labels will not promise to cure particular ailments or conditions.

Educate Yourself

Obtaining good books on herbal remedies must be a priority. No one is going to tell you what you need or prescribe to or for you unless he is a trained doctor or medical herbalist who

WARNING AND DISCLAIMER

I am not a doctor and do not prescribe. The following information is based upon product literature and historical uses of herbs, as well as personal experiences. I strongly suggest that you acquire reliable reference books and firsthand, knowledgeable information from a doctor, naturopathic physician, or herbalist with medicinal background (see resource pages) before embarking on any herbal healing routine either for yourself or for your child. Always use extreme caution when working with unfamiliar herbs.

Ask questions until you are satisfied with the answers. Remember, the only dumb questions are the ones that are not asked.

specializes in herbal healing. These are few and far between. If you find one, employ her by all means. This can often be done by phone if you can accurately describe the child's symptoms and follow verbal directions.

The merits of herbal medicine are confirmed each day be scientific evidence, the holistic community, and families like yours that have experienced what too often seem to be miracles in healing. We can now walk into a health food store or mail-order the preparations a family may have had to labor most of the summer to produce. Herbs have been in use for centuries. There hasn't been a corner drugstore for nearly that long and the drugs that are prescribed every day are often younger than your kids! To take the fear and uncertainty out of using herbal remedies for your family, you must seek as much information as possible. Call companies and ask for educational materials, seek out local practitioners and study groups, and read, read, read. Of course, knowing your child well is the best therapeutic aid any parent has.

Integrating Herbal Care with Your Medical Care

Getting kids to take medicine is a familiar, age-old problem. Herbs can be especially trying to give to kids because some taste yucky to young ones and may be strange-looking and -smelling in their raw forms. The interference from other well-meaning adults can undermine a family's healing choices. I recall very clearly the gut-wrenching decisions I had to make when trying to incorporate herbs into my child care. I was called weird and accused of trying crazy things with my children's health. When children hear these conflicting messages, it is difficult for them also to trust your herbal or alternative-care practices.

I have been lucky enough to find doctors who now accept my personal health-care choices. In fact, my current physician calls me and consults when her patients are using herbs along with prescribed medications. I would never lie to a doctor about my use of herbs with my children because to do so, especially in front of them, would undermine my healing abilities in their eyes. Also, some drugs and herbs may not be compatible, nor may both be needed. Be as open and honest as possible. If you are not comfortable with a certain healthcare practitioner, move on until you find someone whom you can comfortably work with. Remember, you're the one doing the shopping and you will only get what you want by being persistent. (I said persistent not disrespectful or rude.)

Herbs to Know

Herbs with names like echinacea, Oregon grape root, valerian, pleurisy root, feverfew, mullein, astragalus, yarrow, and skullcap may sound unusual. They are, in addition to more common herbs such as catnip, chamomile, garlic, peppermint, fennel, and ginger, some of the mainstays of herbal healing. (See chapter 1 for more detailed information on specific herbs.)

Formulas like Auntie Cham made by Herbs for Kids can be easily understood when the individual herbs are known. Traditionally, skullcap, catnip, hops, chamomile, and fennel are believed to calm the individual. Knowing this, I must assume that Auntie Cham is the formula I want to have in my home to help calm an upset child. Uncle Val is another formula you may want to invite to visit you, containing skullcap, chamomile, valerian, hops, fennel, and catnip formula.

Product Tip
HERBAL REMEDIES

Where were Sunny Mavor and Herbs for Kids (see resource list) when my children were small? I first became aware of this company at Herb Fest '93, an annual meeting and educational weekend sponsored by Frontier Herbs in Iowa every August. There are lectures from practicing herbalists, homeopaths, aromatherapists, manufacturers of natural products, retailers, and just about anyone else who has an interest in herbs to enhance his quality of life. Herbs for Kids offers organic, alcohol-free, high-quality, tasty herbal products for children. If you are new to herbs, this company offers products that would take a tremendous effort to produce on your own while attending to a busy household. Sunny Mavor, a practicing herbalist, also offers a pamphlet called "Herbs for Children" that details the basics of selecting herbs for specific ailments.

When a child is teething Gum-Omile oil may be helpful — for topical use only — with its almond oil, willow bark, chamomile, clove bud oil, and vitamin E formula. I must caution that these formulas are safe because they are in a blend. This does not mean that any of the ingredients are safe to use individually. For instance, I would not suggest that anyone use clove bud oil for teething or toothache, although it is sometimes recommended for this. It is extremely potent and must be used with caution. These formulas take a lot of the guesswork out of using herbs; however, a little knowledge can be dangerous. Please do not try to duplicate such formulas on your own without proper training and guidance. The formula developers should have years of experience behind their wares.

NATURAL HEALTHCARE FOR GROWING CHILDREN

As your child grows, your knowledge of the world of herbs can grow with them. By the time your child is three years old, you can have a working knowledge of some basic herbs, and other remedies that will be of benefit for your household. Children have a natural curiosity and will be eager to know what you are doing to heal them. Be sure to tell them exactly what you're doing and to exercise caution when working with any type of remedy or treatment, natural or otherwise, so they understand that this is careful business that needs to be handled by an adult.

Learn to Understand Their Needs

Communication can become a major part of your helping your children. Listen carefully to them. They may be saying a lot with their behavior, much more than they are able to articulate to you verbally. Watch their moods, preferences, fears, and activity levels. These are all clear indicators of their health. Before they can talk behavior may be your only clue. Watch to see if they are pulling on a sore ear or rubbing a sore spot. Ask them where it hurts and *listen:* with your ears, eyes, and most of all your heart.

DENTAL CARE FOR KIDS

While visiting our dentist (Dr. Mark, as we call him), I asked him what he suggested for tooth care for babies. His recommendation was to use a sterile gauze square and gently wipe away soft plaque from baby's teeth before it can harden. When they're ready for a toothbrush, he recommends very soft bristles so as not to injure the gums. It was formerly believed that a firm toothbrush was best; this view has changed in recent years with more research. He told me that many studies on dental procedures were performed on goats, not humans — how comforting!

Never allow a child to go to sleep or bed for the night with a bottle in his mouth. The liquid pools around the teeth and can lead to decay. Sugar and bacteria team up to destroy teeth.

When you need dental work, bring your child with you. I used to take Christina when she was quite young and allowed her to sit right with me (often right *on* me) while work was being done. I tried to have Dad or someone in the waiting room to take her in case either of our patience wore thin. Take young ones along while older children are being seen. Dr. Mark suggests a child's first visit to the dentist be about 12 to 18 months old.

Be aware of the tooth products your child uses. He needs only the tiniest amount of a toothpaste — just a small dot — although many tubes say add a full strip of toothpaste. Always try to avoid having your child swallowing toothpaste, especially if it contains fluoride. Fluoride may not be as wonderful for children as we thought it was. Do some research into fluoride, and also into any metal materials that are offered as fillings later in life.

We'd love your thoughts . . .

Your reactions, criticisms, things you did or didn't like about this Storey Book. Please use space below (or write a letter if you'd prefer — even send photos!) telling how you've made use of the information . . . how you've put it to work . . . the more details the better! Thanks in advance for your help in building our library of good Storey Books.

Book Title: _____

Purchased From: _____ *Pamela B. Art*

Comments: _____ Publisher, Storey Books

_____

_____

_____

_____

Your Name: _____

Mailing Address: _____

E-mail Address: _____

☐ Please check here if you'd like our latest Storey's Books for Country Living Catalog.

☐ You have my permission to quote from my comments and use these quotations in ads, brochures, mail, and other promotions used to market Storey Books.

Signed _____ Date _____

e-mail–feedback@storey.com   www.storey.com   PRINTED IN THE USA   10/9

From: _____

_____

_____

BUSINESS REPLY MAIL

FIRST-CLASS MAIL   PERMIT NO. 2   POWNAL VT

POSTAGE WILL BE PAID BY ADDRESSEE

STOREY'S BOOKS FOR COUNTRY LIVING
STOREY COMMUNICATIONS INC
RR1 BOX 105
POWNAL VT   05261-9988

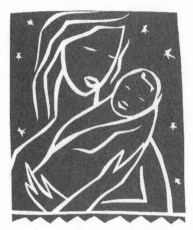

Creating a
Healthy, Welcoming
Environment for
Your Child

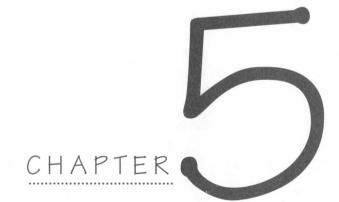

CHAPTER 5

The time you spend preparing for and welcoming your child into the world will come back to you in the form of a well-balanced family system, full of good health and close family ties. Giving our children the best start possible is the least we owe these little ones we welcome into the world. Life can be a challenge and the headstart we instill in our children today may very well be just the added protection they will need in an ever-changing world.

GETTING OFF TO A GOOD BEGINNING

In today's society, more and more people are opting for a better, holistic, natural, organic, and environmentally conscious way of life. I invite you to explore the ways — some ancient and redis-covered — in which you can enhance the relationship between you and your child, children, and society as a whole.

Look around. What do you really need to make your home as baby- and child-friendly as possible? What will it take to bring you and your children a better quality of life? Clean up, let go, and most of all *enjoy* those children. They are ours only to guide. Let's give them the best start possible.

Remember that the time you invest in your children will surely enhance your parent-child relationship. The sense of importance you show them will result in higher self-esteem and much healthier children in body, mind, and spirit. Make your children realize that they are worthy of all the love and care that you bestow upon them; once they believe in you they can begin to believe in themselves. Keep a journal during these early days for both of you to read later in life. Write down your feelings, for they will fade into a new day and you will seldom remember them the same way again.

We can seek alternatives to everyday, corporate, TV-oriented, mass-produced, chemically altered, overmedicated, undereducated, overstimulated, overadvertised, out-of-control, canned, packaged, prompted, and charged-on-credit life. Rais-ing a child in a meaningful, heartfelt way is a challenge to be undertaken with great care. Here are a few practices that may help.

Bless Away

A "bless away" is a rite to prepare for the arrival of a new baby. This is a very personal form of a baby shower, a special event to bless you as a new mother on your journey toward birth. It is a time to be pampered and babied a bit yourself as well as to receive the best wishes of those closest in your life. It is, to me, like a meeting of fairy godmothers, who all bestow a gift upon you and your child. Massage, songs, baths, hair braiding, food preparation, cleaning and helping the mother-to-be get ready for her big day is the focus. When I attend a bless away, I usually give a bottle of labor massage oil redolent of heady jasmine absolute, lavender, and possibly some neroli. Ask which essential oils are a personal favorite of the mother-to-be.

Invite the people the woman truly needs to be able to relax enough to ride the ebb and flow of labor and birth, including relatives, friends, and the father. Or, he may want to set up a bless away of his own with his friends and family. Include any other children the mother-to-be has — a special gift is a nice way to remind them of their importance in this family process.

SHOWER GIFTS

Shower gifts can be anything from well wishes to dish-washing coupons. Be sure to ask the new parents what will be useful to them. What you think they may be able to use may not be their idea of what they need at all. I have often waited to give gifts until a child was born to see what was not received, yet was needed.

Practical supplies shouldn't be overlooked: Diapers, blankets, clothes, and basic baby-care products are always nice to receive. A quality car seat is a must. Several friends can chip in on the cost. A picture-taking session is a great way to remember a friend and a new child. Put photos in a pretty album and give as a memory book. Books or blank journals are always welcome gifts for mothers-to-be.

Herbal Tea Gift Basket

A basket of assorted ready-to-use herbal teas make a useful gift. These could include specialty tea blends such as those made by Traditional Medicinals with names like Mother's Milk, Pregnancy Tea, or Female Toner. Raspberry leaf, chamomile, peppermint, and ginger teas are nice too in tea bag or loose form. If you select the loose form of herbs, include a small tea strainer or tea infuser spoon. Include a cup with a message or artwork particularly appropriate for the expecting mother.

Bath Salts

Mildly scented jars of bath salts are a welcome gift for someone who will probably be too busy to make them herself. While precious oils such as neroli, rose, sandalwood, or jasmine can be so costly, salts extend them. A mere drop of oil can turn a jar of sea salt into a very pleasant experience for both the blender and the receiver. These can be kept on a cool, dark, shelf for those times of need.

Small 1-pint canning jars are great for packaging bath salt gifts. They are usually available at the grocery or hardware store. Simply measure out enough sea salt to fill the jar, then pour it into a bowl, add two to four drops of pure essential oil, and blend well to make sure all the lumps are well crushed and evenly distributed throughout the salts. (See page 58 for essential oil combination recipes.) Add a small amount of rose petals, lavender buds, or sandalwood chips (approximately ¼–½ teaspoon is desired), for color and texture. Please don't dye these salts. Enjoy them naturally. Add a ribbon and an attractive label (including instructions on how to use) and you have a lovely gift.

A Living Gift

Plant a tree — it's a wonderful way to commemorate a birth. A ginkgo tree is a good symbol, because it's the oldest known living tree. This tree with its longevity carries a wish for strength against adversity. It helps to remind a new being on this earth that it's possible to face the odds and come out as glorified as the ancient ginkgo tree. An oak tree is also an ancient symbol of strength; it has been revered and worshiped as such for thousands of years. Encourage the expectant parents to plant the tree in a place where the child will be able to see it grow. In today's mobile society, this isn't always easy, but perhaps you will be able to plant it at a grandparent's home or other familiar, fairly stable place your family frequents.

If each family planted a new tree each time a new child was born, the environmental woes we face with the wanton destruction of trees would be lessened. Think of how ardently these trees would be defended once they have been imbued with this special symbolic meaning — meaning that all trees should naturally have. This would bring a whole new meaning to "The Family Tree."

Potted herb plants that a mother can use for her own and her baby's well-being are also a thoughtful gift.

The Gift of Time

The gift of your love, attention, and time is greatly needed and appreciated. Offer to spend time with the baby's siblings to help them, too, feel special. An I.O.U. for help after baby is home will be a boon to the new mom.

GIFT WRAPPING IDEA

A receiving blanket and baby pins make a great gift wrap. There's no paper and ribbon to throw away. Simply wrap the gift in the blanket and pin it closed.

NAMING YOUR BABY

The name each of us bears has an impact on who we are and what we experience. Having a name that is easy to make fun of is a child's nightmare. Give serious thought to what you will name your child.

When asked what I was going to name my daughter I simply said I had to wait and see who she was. Her dad had liked the name Ina. I contributed Christ after her dawn Good Friday birth; thus, we ended up with Christina. I later received a call from her great-grandmother, who I later found out had the middle name Christina. That was, indeed, my daughter's great-great-grandmother's name!

Look up the meanings of different names. Ask family how the names they use were found. What were some of your ancestors' names? Which names sound good to your ear and feel right with your family name? Write out a possible name and look at the initials. Say the name out loud and even trying spitting it out, middle name included, much like you may need to when being stern with a little one. *The Name Book* by Pierre Le Rouzic is a helpful source (see reading list).

PREPARING SIBLINGS

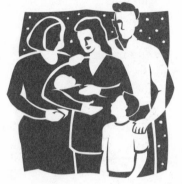

Siblings may have their own little rituals to help ease the adjustment to the changes that come with a new brother or sister. Brothers, sisters, and stepkids need to be able to interact with a new baby. I recall clearly how proud my stepson, David, was of his young sister. He drew pictures of me pregnant and all of us happy and smiling. He was quite worried when I went to the hospital, and was the first one I called when his sister was born. He came to the hospital and had to stand on a box to see her. He was eager to help and I allowed him to do so whenever possible.

With guidance, siblings can be a great help. They must be reminded often that they, too, are special and loved for their own qualities. I am David's stepmother but we never told a lot of folks. We used to smile when people said he looked like me. I am to this day very close to David, as he is to Christina. We share a love and concern for one another that was forged a long time ago when we were all trying to get used to being a family.

Sibling-Building Time

Go to story hour at the library or local bookstore with both baby and sibling to build the sense of shared activities and experiences. Include siblings in massages, baths, and walks to strengthen the sense that you are caring for both of them.

Encourage an older child to take some responsibility for caring for and feeding the younger one, with your supervision. Allow the older one to feel needed and important to the care of their new little brother or sister. Let the older one help you get things ready for baby's bath or massage. And after baby is asleep or with dad, give the sibling the same loving attention that baby receives. Remind children that they were babies once too, and they too needed the care and attention you are now showering on the new baby. Remind them that a baby is helpless and needs the love and care of siblings and parents.

FINDING A SUPPORTIVE COMMUNITY

When you're raising a child naturally, it's very important to find a community of like-minded people whom you can turn to for support, information, and sharing. I have been fortunate to be within 50 miles of many wonderful practitioners of natural healing and lifestyle modalities. You may have these kind of great folks near you too. We all have to live somewhere, and you'd be surprised who may be right in your own backyard. Ask at the doctor's office, church, the hospital, or the library. Word of mouth is the best referral. Be persistent; your children's future is the reward for the diligent work you do to educate yourself.

Seek Out Natural Health Groups

Does your area have a food co-op, a health food store, a whole foods restaurant, an herb shop, a holistic health center? How about a newsletter or play group? If so, go there; ask questions, seek knowledge, get involved in your own and your children's well-being and overall good health.

If you see a child and parents whom you admire or wonder about please, don't hesitate to introduce yourself, and ask them how they learned whatever it is you admire about their relationship. They'll probably be pleased, and will share what they know. And perhaps you'll gain a friendship.

TAKING BABY ALONG: BABY CARRY WRAPS

The practice of wrapping a baby in a fabric carrier to keep her safe and secure without encumbering the parent is ancient and spreads across many cultures. I have friends who adopted their son in Guatamala who received an impromptu "baby-wrapping lesson" at the marketplace by a woman who was a stranger to them. There are a variety of commercial baby-wrapping products available so you can take your baby along as you do your daily activities (see resources on page 147). Try different baby carriers until you find one that works for you.

Help Care for All Children

The maternal/paternal instinct is one of the strongest forces on earth. It is strong, deep, universal, and ageless. It is the force that makes you want the best for children. It is the force that shouts, "Enough!" to the use of dangerous chemicals in our everyday lives. It the force that enables us to go through sometimes unbearable circumstances to aid our child or any child in need.

Today as I worked in my herb and flowerbeds I heard a cry of "Mommy, Mommy, Mommy." I looked to the apartments down the street and saw a young boy of about 3 or 4 in panic as he called for his missing parent. His cries made me instinctually want to help him however I could. The sound clearly touched something deep inside of me.

I believe in the concept "It takes a whole village to raise a child." We all share the responsibility for creating the best and safest environment possible for young children who cross our paths. I would like to feed, cuddle, and teach with love every child in the world.

SURROUND YOUR CHILD WITH HERBS

Herbs, with their natural healing properties and memorable aromas, are a wonderful part of a child's world. Learn to plant and grow herbs, harvest them, and make them part of your family's aromatic mile markers by which you trace the journey of time and the lives of family members. Nurturing a small garden can be much like nurturing a small child. It requires time and attention, yet the rewards are many.

Plant, harvest, and use these "nature's helpers" — they'll impart to you and your family the knowledge of the earth. Growing, gathering, and incorporating herbs and spices into your routines will provide a lifetime of delight. They can enhance everything from your bath to the foods you eat. Herbs provide material for home crafts or gift projects, and, of course, enhance the landscape.

A Simple Herb Garden

There are many wonderful books that include information on design, maintenance, and use of an herb garden. One of my favorites is *Herbal Treasures* by Phyllis Shaudys, which covers many ways to use herbs in daily life, in gardening, as edible flowers, for crafts, body care, aromatherapy, making potpourri, and cooking, to name a few topics from a collection of authors who are herbal treasures (see reading list).

I like to grow what I use and use what I grow; you can do the same. A "simple" is an ancient name for an easy herbal remedy. You can grow the herbs needed to make simples in the form of baths, hair rinses, and facial steams.

HERBS FOR A SIMPLE UTILITARIAN GARDEN

Chamomile (*Matricaria chamomilla*)
Echinacea (*Echinacea angustifolia*)
Lavender (*Lavandula officinalis*)
Lemon balm (*Melissa officinalis*)
Lemon verbena (*Aloysia triphylla*)
Peppermint (*Mentha piperita*)
Rose geranium (*Pelargonium graveolens*)
Rose (*Rosaceae*)
Rosemary (*Rosmarinus officinalis*)
Spearmint (*Mentha spicata*)

BASIC HERBS FOR A COOK'S GARDEN

Basil (*Ocimum basilicum*)
Chives (*Allium schoenoprasum*)
Dill (*Anethum graveolens*)
Lemon basil (*Ocimum basilicum 'Citriodorum'*)
Lemon thyme (*Thymus x citriodorus*)
Parsley (*Petroselinum sativum*)
Rosemary (*Rosmarinus officinalis*)
Sage (*Salvia officinalis*)
Tarragon (*Artemisia dracunculus*)
Thyme (*Thymus vulgaris*)

Many herbs are easily grown, with high yields. Once established, some herbs will thrive for many years and provide you with enough extra to share with fellow gardeners. A small patch of mint (and most gardeners know that no patch of mint ever stays small) can provide enough harvest for lots of tummy-soothing tea. A small patch of chamomile saved Peter Rabbit and could surely soothe any little one who has been frightened and is in need of a peaceful rest. (**Note:** Chamomile has been found to aggravate allergies and hayfever in some people, so be wary of reactions.)

Growing Herbs in Small Spaces

You don't need a large yard to grow nature's pantry goods. Herbs may even be grown indoors in pots or outside on a patio. Some of the nicest herb gardens I've ever visited were on patios or decks. I saw one growing in holes cut in 20-pound bags of potting soil that were cleverly camouflaged with straw. You can grow herbs in almost any improvised container: pots, buckets, coffee cans, even old shoes. Just make sure they've got proper drainage and fertilization. Be creative in adding beauty to the landscaping around your home with herb plantings.

TIPS FOR GARDENING MOTHERS

The gentle exercise and peace of mind you get from tending these precious herbs can be a joy. I used to do a bit of gardening when my daughter was asleep or playing nearby. Gardening and harvesting in early morning or early evening worked best for me and avoided overexposure to the sun's harsh midday rays. The exercise helped me to slowly lose some of the "baby fat" I had gained in pregnancy. Cooking with the fresh and dried herbs helped me to flavor dishes without added fats or salt.

If you are breastfeeding, please research thoroughly the herbs or spices that you take internally as flavoring agents or teas.

Harvesting and Storing Herbs

Fresh herbs give the grower a sense of pride and satisfaction. Harvesting is a great activity to share with a child. It's especially meaningful if you are making herbal remedies: you are allowing the child to be involved with her healing. She also may be more receptive to trying something she had a role in making.

Herbs can be easily harvested by cutting them one-third of the way down the stalk, and then gathering several cut stalks into a bunch and holding with a rubber band. Use an open paperclip to hang each bunch in a place out of direct sunlight. Make sure herbs are very dry; they should hang for about two weeks. Strip dried leaves or flowers off of the stalk and store them in a well-sealed jar, labeled and placed in a dark cupboard. The herbs you harvest in the summer will be your best allies in the winter.

Store dried herb leaves or flowers whole when possible. Wait to crumble them just before brewing the tea or making the remedy because this releases the pure essential oils.

MAKE SURE YOUR HOME IS CHILD-SAFE

Store herbs, oils, and homeopathic remedies well away from little hands. I once taught preschool and the drug companies would ask us to test their childproof bottles with our kids. Usually the children had the bottles open before some of the adults . . . scary! Many natural substances are less harmful than most synthetic drugs; however, extreme caution must always be observed. I have heard of children drinking tinctures — the alcohol in them causes most of the problems they experienced. Some pure essential oils can be toxic and their use must be supervised at all times.

Never, ever suggest that herbs, oils, or homeopathic remedies are candy. This could confuse a child. Explain that some herbs are for beverages and some for medicine. Learn something about the wild herbs — weeds to many — you'll then be able to show a little one which plants are good and which ones should be avoided altogether. Never give a child the impression that all plants are good or edible. They must be cautioned *never* to touch or taste any plant without you or another responsible adult present.

If you are going to eat herbs and/or edible flowers, be careful in front of children. Perhaps wait until they are old enough to distinguish plant foods from nonedible types. Teach them to limit plant foods to those that come directly from your hand or that of a trusted instructor or family member. Remind them never to eat or encourage another child to eat any plant, fruit, flower, berry, bark, or grass that has not been directly offered by and explained to them by you or a trusted adult.

Explain to children about each and every plant. They *must* know some are *not* to be touched or eaten! Label plants properly. A good plant identification book is valuable; it would make a great baby shower or bless away gift. I like *Baby-Safe Houseplants and Cut Flowers: A Guide to Keeping Children and Plants Safely Under the Same Roof* by John I. Alber and Delores M. Alber (see reading list).

AVOID PLANT POISONING

In the book *Baby-Safe Houseplants and Cut Flowers*, John and Delores Alber list the five most important steps to eliminate risks of plant poisoning:

1. Identify your plants.
2. Learn which plants are poisonous, and which are not.
3. Display plants safely.
4. Teach your children never to eat nonfood plants.
5. Be prepared for emergencies. Label, label, label!

I would add to this list: Know your poison control number. Have it posted so that other household members, sitters, or guests have clear access to it. If you have a plant — in the garden or in the house — and you don't know what it is, check with your local Cooperative Extension Service, master gardener hotline, or local plant nursery. They can aid in plant identification. Even if your child is only a baby, she will grow right along with that no-name plant in its welcome home planter that you forgot about until your two-year-old munched on some.

HOUSEPLANT SAFETY

Be just as cautious about the safety of common houseplants in your home as you are about the herbs you grow. Here are a few to be aware of:

Toxic Household Plants
Azalea (Rhododendron x hybridum)
Bittersweet (Celastrus scandens)
Holly (Ilex opaca)
Mother-in-law's-tongue (Sansevieria trifasciata)
Philodendron (Philodendron scandens and all Philodendron genus)
Potato: white leaves, eyes, and stems (Solanum tuberosum)

Can Cause Nausea or Discomfort
Amaryllis (Hippeastrum x hybridum)
Gardenia (Gardenia jasminoides)
Poinsettia (Euphorbia pulcherrima)

Reasonably Safe Plants
Boston fern (Nephrolepis exaltata)
Hen-and-chickens or houseleek (Sempervivum tectorum)
Polka-dot plant (Hypoestes phyllostachya)
Rose geranium (Pelargonium graveolens)
Rubber plant (Ficus elastica)
Spider plant (Chlorophytum comosum)
Wandering Jew (Tradescantia fluminensis)
Zebra plant (Aphelandra squarrosa)

Findings Inconclusive/Keep Out of Reach of Children
African violet (Saintpaulia ionantha)
Aloe vera (Aloe barbadensis)
Jade (Crassula argentea)

Bulbs are easily mistaken for food by small children. Store well away from little ones at all times. Make sure these are planted deep in the garden so a child doesn't dig them up.

Keep in mind that the vase water from various cut flowers, like my favorite lily-of-the-valley, can become very toxic. Keep it away from children.

It may be helpful to limit the kinds of plants you grow. Definitely know all their names. If a child should ever eat a plant, try to bring a piece of it with you to the hospital or be able to give an accurate description to a poison-control official.

The same holds true for any remedy a child may get a hold of or any insect that has stung or animal that has bitten him. Knowing what they are dealing with is more than half the battle for an emergency team.

Keep syrup of ipecac and activated charcoal on hand in case of an accidental ingestion of a potentially toxic plant material. Always check with poison control before administering either of these remedies. Syrup of ipecac is most effective when given as soon as possible after ingestion of potentially toxic material.

If you have a loved one who is expecting or living with young children, send her this information. Look around the local day-care center. Does it have plants? Are they safe? How about your sitter's home? Or your relatives' where a young child might stay while you're away? Restaurants, offices, parks, playgrounds all have the potential to harbor toxic plants. Be aware, be educated.

Especially if you are going to use herbs or essential oils in your home, information on toxicity is of the utmost importance. The time you invest could prevent a tragedy. The Herb Research Foundation (see resource list) can also provide useful information.

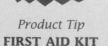

Product Tip
FIRST AID KIT

The *Perfectly Safe Company* specializes in child safety products (see resource list). I highly recommend purchasing a first aid kit to keep in your home. You will be able to enjoy the company of safe houseplants and have peace of mind.

KIDS AND BUGS

Bugs! Who needs them? Who wants them? Kids do! Most kids have a fascination for these often tiny creatures — some adults, too, I might add!

My friend Phil has an unusual preference in his diet. He eats bugs. He has shocked and amazed children on more than one occasion in my herb gardens. They stand and watch, dumbfounded, as Phil delightfully dines among the colorful, fragrant herbs and flowers. Yes, I know this sounds disgusting, even unthinkable. However, the fact is that man has enjoyed crawly cuisine for centuries. Some bugs, such as bees and ants, can actually bite back or sting after they have died!

The point of this information is to help you not to bug out if your little one decides to dine with a cricket, or on one. Write to a poison control center for a list of insects and their toxicity, or lack thereof. Always try to obtain a sample of any insect ingested by your child for proper identification. Buy a bug book and familiarize yourself and your children with the pros and cons of coexisting with bugs.

Watching bugs, worms, and small animals offer many opportunities to interact with our children. Sit still and watch a butterfly (or "flutter-by," as I refer to it). Marvel at how it goes from flower to flower, or how a yellow-pollen-coated bee works his day away to ensure his survival.

Natural Insect Control in Your Yard

I have always encouraged bees in my yard and gardens, and have never had any problems with stings — for me or for others — but I must admit that spiders have given me a run for my money. The poisoning of any insects would cost me the beneficial ones in the process. Praying mantises delight the children who visit, and butterflies seem to spend a lot of time here. I remember so many more kinds of butterflies when I was young, though; perhaps too many butterfly collections were made. I let milkweed grow freely in a section of my yard to feed the monarchs as they pass through on their migration to Mexico. (This grew out of a report Christina did in grade school on monarchs.)

Children have told me many times that I have the coolest bugs in my yard. Adults often comment that they see insects here that they have never seen elsewhere. I attribute this to the fact that no insecticides have been used on this property for at least the 17 years that I have lived and gardened here. My small corner of the earth seems to grow in harmony and I was never worried about letting the children play freely at any time. When visitors ask what I am going to do about an obvious pest problem on a plant, I usually reply, "Plant some more so there is enough for us both the bugs and us."

Always be careful with herbicides or any "-cides" you encounter or consider using. Companion planting — putting garlic and other repellant-type seedlings around plants that tend to draw bugs — is worth exploring. I have garlic, garlic chives, common chives, and onions planted all around my roses to help stem the flow of beetles. I simply pull apart cloves of garlic and plant them around the plants I would like protected. Heck, if it works against vampires, how do bugs stand a chance? The ones that attack my plants are picked off by hand. That's how I test the mettle of new work-study students: If you get past the beetle-picking project, you're in.

AVOID LAWN PESTICIDES, AS WELL

In addition to limiting the pesticides that go into your children's bodies, beware of pesticides that may get on their bodies. Use caution when employing chemical lawn services. I have seen babies and children playing on freshly treated lawns, with the little warning flags still flying in the wind. Be alert to chances of your children accidentally being exposed to pesticides and chemical fertilizers.

Homeopathic Remedies for Insect Bites and Stings

Homeopathic Apis is something I keep nearby in case of insect stings. *SSStop Sting,* a homeopathic gel, is useful, too. My daughter once stepped in a bee's nest in the field across the street. I put her in the tub with an armful of fresh basil *(Ocimum basilicum)* from the garden. Her welts went down in a few hours, and she was much better. You can smash up fresh plantain *(Plantago major)* and apply it directly to a sting or bite. Ice often helps me initially to relieve the pain. Tea tree and lavender essential oils dabbed on stings and bites will soothe too.

Safe and Effective Insect Repellents

Repelling insects from the immediate area is an international pastime. We are constantly trying to conquer this natural cohabitant of the earth. I try to coexist with these little creatures, but there are certainly times when I wish they would go somewhere else to play. When a mosquito is buzzing in my ear as I try to drop off to sleep, I don't exactly appreciate his song.

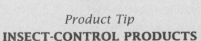

Product Tip
INSECT-CONTROL PRODUCTS

Green Ban (see resource list) contains no animal products, petrochemicals, alcohol, solvents, artificial perfumes, cortisone, dyes, or sometimes irritating citrus oils.

Green Ban products contain citronella, peppermint, myrrh, bergaptene-free bergamot (bergaptene is the constituent in bergamot essential oil that is believed to cause the pigment in skin to darken unevenly), tea tree, calendula, mint, and other natural, nontoxic ingredients. They have had quite a time marketing their products. It seems the Environmental Protection Agency (EPA) has a bit to learn about natural insect products. Contact the company for its informative free brochure. It offers Green Ban For Pets, Green Ban For People, and Double Strength Green Ban For People. Green Ban For Plants is sadly in limbo at the present time; however, this recipe is offered in its stead.

GREEN BAN'S HOMEMADE PLANT SPRAY

1 teaspoon finely chopped garlic
1½ teaspoons soy or corn oil
1 cup water
¼ cup buttermilk
¼ teaspoon mild liquid soap
2 teaspoons liquid kelp
½ teaspoon eucalyptus pure essential oil

Put first four ingredients into blender and blend well for 2 minutes. Add the liquid soap and liquid kelp. Blend well for 1 minute. Decant into a large measuring container. Top up with water to 2-quart mark. Add ½ teaspoon eucalyptus pure essential oil. Stir. Strain through cloth. Use undiluted. Perishable.

Makes 2 quarts

In Australia, where these products originated, a "green ban" is a citizens ban on projects and products that are detrimental to the future of plants, animals, and people. You can make a difference, too!

Some of the herbal and aromatherapy bug-repellant creations include aromatic essential oils known for their insect-repelling qualities, specifically patchouli, rosemary, lavender, citronella, red cedarwood, and eucalyptus. These are diluted in soy and canola base oils. The scent of some essential oils will repel bugs, even when they are not applied directly to the skin. I once put cotton balls with a drop of peppermint and rose geranium pure essential oils in the pockets of the members of a Brownie troop that I was taking on a plant tour through the woods. Or, you can make a spray repellent to apply to your hat and clothes.

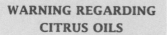

WARNING REGARDING CITRUS OILS

Some citrus oils can be irritating to the skin when used in too strong a dilution. They can also be photosensitive and cause irritation upon exposure to the sun.

Household Bugs

If you have animals and are combating a recurring flea or tick problem, there is a natural deterrent. Sweet orange pure essential oil provides an effective deterrent to pests when mixed with lavender essential oil and used in borax as a carpet freshener or in water as a spray on rugs and upholstered furniture.

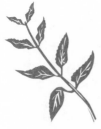

BUG REPELLENT SPRAY

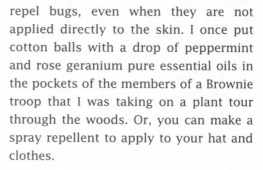

8 drops of a combination of peppermint and
rose geranium pure essential oils
4 ounces of water

Combine the essential oils and water in a small 4-ounce spray bottle. Spray clothing and exposed skin, avoiding areas around the eyes, mouth, and nose. The peppermint will help cool you off on a hot day, as well. I often spray my hat to keep little buddies from buzzing around my skin. Be sure to wash your hands after handling pure essential oils so they do not come into contact with eyes or mouth. And, as always, remember that less is best; only a drop or two (or a quick spray) is ever needed.

FLEA AND TICK CARPET FRESHENER

15 drops sweet orange essential oil
10 drops lavender essential oil
2 cups borax

Mix well, making sure the little lumps of essential oils are well distributed. Sprinkle this on carpet and let stand for at least an hour, then vacuum. As a bonus, your sweeper will smell nice, and this will also prevent insects from breeding in the carpet-cleaner bag.

If you prefer a spray, combine the essential oils with at least 8 ounces of water in a spray bottle. Apply this sweet smell to curtains, furniture, and rugs to suggest to little bugs that they go elsewhere. Keep these mixtures out of the reach of children and well labeled, as you should all of your homemade products. Also record the date prepared, as essential oil mixtures don't have a very long shelf life. Use them as soon as possible.

Head Lice

Head lice can be a problem for older toddlers and school-age children. If you've ever had to deal with this common condition, you know how difficult and distasteful it can be to treat. Essential oils make a much nicer alternative to chemical pesticides. Here is a recipe that originally appeared in my book, *The Essential Oils Book.*

OIL TREATMENT FOR HEAD LICE

10 drops each of rosemary, lavender, rose geranium,
and eucalyptus essential oils
2 ounces sweet almond oil (as base)

Combine the essential oils with the base oil and mix well. Rub oil throughout hair and leave treatment on for at least 1 hour. Apply shampoo and rinse hair well. Comb the hair with a nit comb after shampooing. Repeat the procedure in a few days.

Be very careful when applying oil near eyes. If essential oil gets in the eyes, wipe it out with plain sweet almond oil, not water. The water can disperse the oil too quickly.

CLOSING

As I sit here peacefully looking out my window, I watch Mrs. Squirrel giving nest-building lessons to her young. Animals, like humans, have forged a trust with their young. This trust is the foundation of their survival, and also of ours. In closing, I ask you to keep this in mind each time you are momentarily tempted or overcome to the point where you could belittle, injure, hurt, or lie to a child; any child. It is this breach of trust between adult and child that has broken the bonds that are so necessary for survival and for the ability to give and receive trust.

When coping seems impossible, take time out! Take a deep breath or two and **think**! Call a friend, a relative, family, neighbor or help line and if none of them are there for you, call upon yourself — your higher self, the will deep inside. Use nature's helpers — Bach flower remedies, homeopathic medicines, pure essential oils, herb teas, rosewater, a bath, or a walk — to aid you on the journey through parenthood.

It is our own growing up that often makes raising children such a challenge. At various ages we re-experience anniversary reactions that are usually unconscious in nature yet play a very real and concrete role in our day-to-day interactions with others, especially our children. Make a vow not to perpetuate negative behavior. It takes great bravery and perseverance not only to raise a child, but to raise him or her above your own limitations, or perceived ones.

Just as I know Mrs. Squirrel will teach her babies to build a proper nest, I know you and I can teach our babies, too. I wish you all the love and nurturance of a mother's heart, the peace of a slumbering child, and the joy of living.

RESOURCE LIST

The organizations and companies listed here are just a few of the many resources you will find once you start exploring. Be sure to look for groups and stores in your own community that offer these or similar services and products. When you contact one of the following groups, please tell them where you found them and let them know you are glad they are there.

ALTERNATIVE MEDICINE ORGANIZATIONS

American Association of Holistic Healing Centers
109 Holly Crescent, Suite 201
Virginia Beach, VA 23451
(804) 422-9033

American Association of Naturopathic Physicians
2366 Eastlake Avenue East
Seattle, WA 98102
(206) 323-7610

American Holistic Medical Association
4101 Lake Boone Trail, Suite 201
Raleigh, NC 27607
(919) 787-5181

John Bastry College of Applied Kinesiology
P.O. Box 905
Lawrence, KS 66044-0905
(913) 542-1801

Nurse Healers Professional Association
234 Fifth Avenue, Suite 3399
New York, NY 10001

AROMATHERAPY SUPPLIES

Aroma Vera
5901 Rodeo Drive
Los Angeles, CA 90016-4312
(800) 669-9514
Marcel Lavabre, ext. 10

Aromaland Inc.
1326 Rufina Circle
Santa Fe, NM 87505
(800) 933-5267

Aromatherapy for Kids
18347 Sherman Way
Reseda, CA 91335
(800) 955-8253

Aura Cacia
P.O. Box 399
Weaverville, CA 96093
(800) 437-3301

The Essential Oil Company
P.O. Box 206
Lake Oswego, OR 97034
(800) 729-5912

Herbal Endeavours Ltd.
3618 S. Emmons Avenue
Rochester Hills, MI 48307-5621
(248) 852-0796
Colleen K. Dodge
Catalog $2.00. Colleen is available for lectures, book signings, and workshops.

Hydrosols
Video Remedies, Inc.
P.O. Box 290866
Davie, FL 33329-0866
(800) 733-4874

Star Power Essentials
680 Dickinson Avenue
Ben Lomond, CA 95005
(408) 336-5828; (800) 457-0904

AROMATHERAPY ORGANIZATIONS

International Federation of Aromatherapists
46 Dal Keith Road
West Dalwich
London SE 21 8LS, England

International Society of Professional Aromatherapists
41 Leicester Road
Hinkley
Leicestershire LE10 1LW,
England
Natural child-care supplies.

BACH FLOWER REMEDIES

The Edward Bach Centre
Mt. Vernon
Bidwell, Wallingford
Oxon OX10 0P2 England

Ellon Bach USA Inc.
P.O. Box 320
Woodmere, NY 11598
(516) 593-2206

Nelson Bach USA Ltd.
1007 W. Upsal Street
Philadelphia, PA 19119
(800) 314-2224
Flower essences brochure.

BREASTFEEDING SUPPORT

Breastfeeding National Network
24-hour help line: (800) 835-5968

CHILD AND FAMILY HEALTH

Feingold Association of the United States
P.O. Box 6550
Alexandria, VA 22306
(703) 768-3287
Information on proper nutrition and its role in health, behavior, and learning.

CHILD SAFETY

The National Child Passenger Safety Association
P.O. Box 841
Ardmore, PA 19003
(202) 939-4993

National Poison Control Center
Georgetown University Hospital
3800 Reservoir Road NW
Washington, DC 20007
(202) 625-6073

National SAFE KIDS Campaign
111 Michigan Avenue NW
Washington, DC 20010-2970
(215) 525-4610

Perfectly Safe Company
7245 Whipple Avenue NW
North Canton, OH 44720
Child-safe products, including first aid kits.

HERBAL PRODUCTS

Country Comfort Herbal Products
288537 Nuevo Valley Drive
Nuevo, CA 92567
(909) 928-4038
Line of natural baby products.

Earth Baby
776-B North Highland Avenue
Atlanta, GA 30306
(404) 607-1656
http://www.mindspring.com/
~ebaby/home.htm

Frontier Co-op Herbs
3021 78th Street
P.O. Box 299
Norway, IA 52318
(800) 669-3275

Herb-Pharm
P.O. Box 116
Williams, OR 97544
(503) 846-6262

Herbs Etc.
1340 Rufina Circle
Santa Fe, NM 87505
(888) 433-1212
Daniel Gagnon, President
Liquid herbal extracts.

Herbs For Kids
151 Evergreen Drive, Suite D
Bozeman, MT 59715
(406) 587-0180; (800) 735-0299

Nature's Products
20020 Conant
Detroit, MI 48234
(313) 891-3900
Gary Wanttaja
*Dried herbs, essential oils, homeo-
pathic remedies, books.*

HOMEOPATHY AND HERBAL MEDICINE

American Botanical Council
P.O. Box 201660
Austin, TX 78720-8868
(512) 331-8868

Boericke and Tafel, Inc.
1011 Arch Street
Philadelphia, PA 19107
(215) 922-2967
Supplier of homeopathic remedies.

Boiron-Barneman
1208 Amosland Road
Norwood, PA 19074
(215) 532-2035

Herb Research Foundation
1007 Pearl Street, Suite 200
Boulder, CO 80302
(303) 449-2265
*Support research and produces
publications on safety of
medicinal herbs.*

**Homeopathic Academy of
Naturopathic Physicians**
4072 9th Avenue NE
Seattle, WA 98015
(206) 547-9665

**Homeopathic Educational
Services**
2124 Kittredge Street
Berkeley, CA 94706
(510) 649-0294; (800) 359-9051

**The International Foundation
for Homeopathy**
2124 Kittredge Street
Berkeley, CA 94704
(510) 649-8930
*Herbal medicine/homeopathic
remedies.*

Standard Homeopathic Company
P.O. Box 61604
436 West Eighth Street
Los Angeles, CA 90014
(213) 321-4284
Supplier of homeopathic remedies.

INFANT AND CHILD PRODUCTS

Audio-Therapy Innovations, Inc.
P.O. Box 550
Colorado Springs, CO 80901
(800) 537-7748

Baby Trekker
Pettersen Infant Products
189 Dadson Row
Flin Flon, Manitoba R8A 0C8,
    Canada
(800) 665-3957

Babyworks
11725 N.W. West Road #2
Portland, OR 97229
(800) 422-2910
Music/recordings.

Cascade Health Care Products
141 Commercial Street, NE
Salem, OR 97301
(800) 443-9942
Catalog carries hooded bath towels.

The Natural Baby Company
816 Silvia Street, 800 B-S
Trenton, NJ 08628-3299
(609) 771-9233

The Relaxation Company
P.O. Box 304
Roslyn, NY 11576
(800) 788-6670
relaxco@aol.com
Produce "Relax and Enjoy Your
    Baby," *tapes by Sylvia Klein Olkin.*

Simple Alternatives
10513 S.E. 30th Street
Bellevue, WA 98004
(800) 735-2082
*Offers 100% cotton diapers, diaper
    supplies, washable nursing pads.*

Weleda
175 North Route 9W
Congers, NY 10920
(914) 268-8572
*Some of the best baby products
    you can find.*

INSECT CONTROL

Green Ban Products
Mulgum Hollow Farm
P.O. Box 146
Norway, IA 52318
(319) 446-7495

MASSAGE ORGANIZATIONS

Renee Gauthier LMT CCE
c/o Irenes Myomassology Institute
18911 W. 10 Mile Road
Southfield, MI 48075
(810) 569-4263

**International Association of
    Infant Massage Instructors**
P.O. Box 16103
Portland, OR 97216
(503) 253-9977

Natal Kneads
Patricia B. Smith RN BSN CTM
21890 8 1/2 Mile Road
Southfield, MI 48075
(810) 354-9047

NATURAL MENSTRUAL CARE

Feminine Options
N14397 380th Street
Ridgeland, WI 54763
(715) 455-1652; (800) 236-4941
*Design, manufacture, and
    distribute* Comfort Curves —
    cloth menstrual lingerie.

Many Moons
Box 59-1594 Fairfield Road
Victoria, BC V8S 1GO, Canada
(604) 592-8815
*Offers line of alternative
    menstrual care products.*

NUTRITION AND FOOD
SAFETY ORGANIZATIONS

Americans for Safe Food
1501 16th Street NW
Washington, DC 20036
(202) 332-9110

**Mothers and Others for
    Pesticide Limits**
40 West 20th Street
New York, NY 10011
(212) 727-2700

ORGANIC FOODS (MAIL ORDER)

Earth's Best Baby Food
4840 Pearl East Circle, Suite 201E
Boulder, CO 80301
(800) 442-4221
*For information on where to find
Earth's Best products call (800)
442-4221. By calling you'll receive
a free subscription to Earth's Best's
parenting newsletter.*

Lundberg Farms
P.O. Box 369
Rockvale, CA 95974
(916) 882-4551

Mountain Ark Trading Company
120 South East Avenue
Fayetteville, AR 72701
(800) 643-8909

Walnut Acres
Walnut Farms Road
Penns Creek, PA 17862
(717) 837-0601

PARENTING SUPPORT ORGANIZATIONS

Active Parenting
810 Franklin Court, Suite B
Marietta, GA 30067
(800) 825-0060

Informed Birth and Parenting Book Service
Box 3675
Ann Arbor, MI 48106
(313) 662-6857
*Publish pamphlet on informed
homebirth options with list of
midwives; $1.00.*

La Leche League International
Box 4079
Schaumburg, IL 60168-4079
(800) La-Leche; (708) 519-7730;
(708) 519-0035 (fax)
http://www.prairienet.org/llli

National Committee for Prevention of Child Abuse
P.O. Box 2866
Chicago, IL 60690
(312) 663-3520

PREGNANCY SUPPORT SERVICES

American College of Nurse-Midwives
1000 Vermont Avenue NW
Washington, DC 20005
(202) 728-9860

Better Beginnings Midwifery Services and Belly Masks
1096 Hartland
Troy, MI 48083
(810) 689-5289
Lisa Forester
BETBEGIN@aol.com
Belly Masks.

Childbirth Education Association
P.O. Box 20852
Milwaukee, WI 53220
(414) 937-5232

Citizens for Midwifery (CFM)
P.O. Box 82227
Athens, GA 30608-2227
(316) 267-7236
http://pages.prodigy.com/www.
cfm.org

Healthy Mothers, Healthy Babies Coalition
409 12th Street SW
Washington, DC 20024-2188
(202) 863-2458; (800) 673-8444

Informed Homebirth/Informed Birth Parenting (IH/IBP) now known as Association of Labor Assistants and Childbirth Educators (ALACE)
P.O.Box 382724
Cambridge, MA 02238
(617) 441-2500
http:www.alace.org
*Trainers of childbirth educators and
birth assistants.*

International Childbirth Education Association (ICEA)
P.O. Box 20048
Minneapolis, MN 55420
(612) 854-8660
They have wonderful "position" papers and statements including a Pregnant Women's Bill of Rights.

Midwifery Today
P.O. Box 2672
Eugene, OR 97402
(800) 743-0974; (514) 344-7438
Jan Tritton, Editor
Midwifery@aol.com
Wonderful publication and listings of conferences and networking opportunities.

Midwives Alliance of North America (MANA)
P.O.Box 175
Newton, KS 67114
MANAinfo@aol.com
http://www.mana.org
(316) 283-4543

Ina May Gaskin, President
41, The Farm
Summertown, TN 38483
Midwife/M@aol.com
Author of Spiritual Midwifery.

National Association of Parents and Professionals for Safe Alternatives in Childbirth (NAPSAC)
Rt. 1, Box 646
Marble Hill, MO 63764
(314) 238-2010
They have a through directory of providers.

Positive Pregnancy and Parenting Fitness
c/o Be Healthy, Inc.
51 Salt Rock Road
Baltic, CT 06330
(203) 822-8573; (800) 433-5523

PUBLICATIONS

Birth Gazette
42-M The Farm
Summertown, TN 38483
(615) 964-3798

Herbs for Health, and **The Herb Companion**
Interweave Press Inc.
201 East Fourth Street
Loveland, CO 80537-5655
(800) 645-3675

Mothering Magazine
P.O. Box 1690
Santa Fe, NM 87504-9774
(800) 984-8116

Susun Weed, Herbalist
Ash Tree Publishing
P.O. Box 64
Woodstock, NY 12498
(914) 246-8081
Publishes books on using herbs in women's healthcare.

SUGGESTED READING

BOOKS

Albers, John I. and Delores M. *Baby-Safe Houseplants & Cut Flowers.* Pownal, VT: Storey Communications, Inc., 1993.

Apple, Rima D. *Mothers & Medicine: A Social History of Infant Feeding, 1890–1950.* Madison, WI: University of Wisconsin Press, 1987.

Armstrong, Liz and Adrienne Scott. *Whitewash: Exposing the Health and Environmental Dangers of Women's Sanitary Products and Disposable Diapers.* Toronto: HarperCollins, 1993.

Baker, Jeannine P. *Prenatal Yoga and Natural Birth.* Berkeley, CA: North Atlantic Press, 1986.

Byers, Dorie. *Natural Body Basics: Making Your Own Cosmetics.* Bargersville, IN: Gooseberry Hill Publications, Inc., 1996.

Cavitch, Susan Miller. *The Natural Soap Book.* Pownal, VT: Storey Publishing, 1995.

Dodt, Colleen K. *The Essential Oils Book.* Pownal, VT: Storey Publishing, 1995.

Dye, Jane. *Aromatherapy for Women and Children, Pregnancy and Childbirth.* England: C.W. Daniel Co., Ltd., 1992.

Earle, Liz. *Illustrated Natural Beauty: A Practical Step-by-Step Guide to Making Lotions, Balms, Tonics.* New York, NY: Random House Value, 1996.

England, Allison. *Aromatherapy for Mother & Baby: Natural Healing with Essential Oils During Pregnancy & Early Motherhood.* Rochester, VT: Inner Traditions, 1993.

Fawcett, Margaret. *Aromatherapy for Pregnancy and Childbirth.* England: Element Books, Ltd., 1993.

Gagnon, Daniel O. *Liquid Herbal Drops In Everyday Use* (booklet). Santa Fe, NM: Santa Fe Botanical Research & Educational Project, 1993.

Gardner, Joy. *The New Healing Yourself Natural Remedies for Adults and Children.* Freedom, CA: The Crossing Press, 1989.

Keller, Erich. *Aromatherapy Handbook for Beauty, Hair, & Skin Care.* Rochester, VT: Inner Traditions, 1991.

Knight, Karin and Jeannie Lumley. *The Baby Cookbook: A Complete Guide to Nutrition, Feeding, and Cooking for Babies Six Months to Two Years of Age.* New York, NY: William Morrow, 1985.

La Leche League International Staff. *The Womanly Art of Breastfeeding.* New York, NY: Penguin, 1991.

Lac, Janet Zand OMD, Rachel Walton RN, and Bob Roundtree, MD. *Smart Medicine for a Healthier Child: A Practical A–Z Reference to Natural and Conventional Treatments for Infants and Children.* United States: Avery Publishing Group, 1994.

Lawless, Julia. *Lavender Oil: The New Guide to Nature's Most Versatile Remedy.* San Francisco, CA: Thorsons, 1995.

———*Rose Oil.* San Francisco: HarperCollins, 1996.

Leboyer, Frederick. *Inner Beauty, Inner Light.* New York: A. Knopf, 1978.

Mothering Magazine. "Immunizations." Santa Fe, NM: John Muir Publications, 1986.

LeRouzic, Pierre. *The Name Book.* Fairfield, IA: Sunstar Publications, 1995.

Mandell, Frederick. *Dr. Mandell's 5-Day Allergy Relief System.* New York, NY: Pocket Books, 1979.

McIntyre, Anne. *The Herbal for Mother and Child.* Rockport, MA: Element, 1992.

Muryn, Mary. *Water Magic: Healing Bath Recipes for the Body, Spirit, & Soul.* New York, NY: Simon & Schuster, 1995.

Natural Choices Company Staff. *The Nontoxic Baby: Reducing Harmful Chemicals from Your Baby's Life.* Twin Lakes, WI: Lotus Press, 1991.

Neustaedter, Randall. *The Immunization Decision: A Guide For Parents.* Berkeley, CA: North Atlantic Books, 1990.

Pottkotter, Louis. *The Natural Nursery: The Parent's Guide to Ecologically Sound, Nontoxic, Safe & Healthy Baby Care.* Chicago, IL: Contemporary Books, 1994.

Riggs, Maribeth. *The Scented Bath.* New York, NY: Penguin, 1991.

Roberts, Margaret. *A Herbal Approach to Pregnancy and Baby Care.* New Zealand: Jonathan Ball Publishers, 1992.

Romm, Aviva Jill. *Natural Healing for Babies and Children.* Freedom, CA: The Crossing Press, 1996.

Sanderson, Liz. *How to Make Your Own Herbal Cosmetics.* New Canaan, CT: Keats Publishing, 1974.

Santillo, Humbart. *Natural Healing with Herbs.* Prescott Valley, AZ: Holm Press, 1987.

Schneider, Vimala. *Infant Massage: A Handbook for Loving Parents.* New York, NY: Bantam Books, 1989.

Shaudys, Phyllis. *Herbal Treasures.* Pownal, VT: Garden Way Publishing, 1990.

Sinclair, Marybetts. *Massage for Healthier Children.* Oakland, CA: Wingbow Press, 1992.

Stillerman, Elaine, LMT. *Mother Massage.* Dell Publishing, 1992.

Tisserand, Maggie. *Aromatherapy for Women.* Rochester, VT: Inner Traditions, 1996.

Tourles, Stephanie. *The Herbal Body Book.* Pownal, VT: Storey Publishing, 1994.

Ullman, Dana, M.P.H. *Homeopathic Medicine for Children and Infants.* NY: G.P. Putnam's Sons, 1992.

Wallerstein, Edward. *Circumcision: An American Health Fallacy.* New York: Springer Publishing, 1980.

Watson, Franzesca. *Aromatherapy Blends and Remedies: Over 800 Recipes for Everyday Use.* London, England: Thorsons, 1995.

Weed, Susan. *Wise Woman Herbal for the Childbearing Years.* Woodstock, NY: Ash Tree Publishing, 1985.

Weiner, Michael A., Ph.D. *Maximum Immunity: How to Fortify Your Natural Defenses.* Boston: Houghton Mifflin Co., 1986.

Ya-li, Fan. *Chinese Pediatric Massage Therapy: A Parent's and Practitioner's Guide to the Treatment and Prevention of Childhood Disease.* Boulder, CO: Blue Poppy Press, 1994.

INDEX

Premenstrual symptoms, remedies
for, 22, 70
Pulsatilla, 37

Rashes, remedy for, 37
Raspberry, 64, 68
Recipes
   baby foods, 116–118
   balms, 97–100
   bath salts, 58–59
   diaper soak, 93
   hair care, 75–76, 91–92
   insect control, 142–143
   massage oils, 47
   potpourri, 80
   room scents, 87
   skin care, 72–73, 104
   tincture, 103
Recycling
   baby food jars, 112
   clothing, 94
"Relax and Enjoy Your Baby"
   (Olkin), 66
Relaxation
   conception and, 41–42
   herb for, 14
   tapes for, 66
Respiratory system, remedies for,
   22–23
Rhus toxicodendron, 37
Rock rose, 38
Rose, 21, 23, 24, 71
Rose geranium, 45, 71
Rosemary, 21, 23, 71
Rosenstone, Maria, 52–53
Rose otto, 82
Rosewater, 81

Sage, 21, 64, 68, 71
Salves. *See* Balms
Sandalwood, 23
Scents
   importance of, 78–80
   room, 84–87
Scrapes, remedy for, 24
Shampoo, 91–92
Siblings, newborns and, 130–131
Simmer pots, 28, 84
Skin care. *See also specific condition*
   aromatic waters for, 81–83

balms, 96–98
carrier oils for, 25, 26
essential oils for, 22–23
herbal tisanes for, 83–84
herbs for, 71
ready-made products for,
   96–98, 101
recipes for, 72–73, 76
Sleep, 106–107
Smith, Patricia B., 49
Sore throat, remedies for, 13, 36, 38
Spearmint, 15, 71
Spice necklace, making, 13
St.-John's-wort, 102–103
Star of Bethlehem, 38
Star Power Essentials, 29, 86
Stomach flu, remedy for, 35
Stomach upset, remedies for, 12,
   13, 14, 15
Stress, remedies for, 24, 42
Stretch marks, preventing, 48–50
Sulphur, 38
Sunburn, remedy for, 22

Tai chi, 53
Teas, herbal, 9–10, 51, 67–68, 128.
   See also Tisanes
Tea tree, 84
Teething, remedies for, 36, 123
Tinctures, 102–103
Tisanes, 83–84
Trees, as gifts, 128–129
Turmeric, 115
Twigg, Vanessa, 42–43

Uncle Val herbal formula, 122

Virus, remedy for, 14
Vutetakis, George, 115–119

Wanttaja, Gary, 98
Weiner, Michael A., 16
Weleda, Inc., 101
Wheat germ oil, 26
Wintergreen, 21, 101
Woodford, Terry, 106–107

Yoga, 52–53